The Consumer's Guide To Nursing Research:

Exercises, Learning Activities, Tools and Resources

The Consumer's Guide To Nursing Research:
Exercises, Learning Activities, Tools and Resources

by

**Holly Skodol Wilson,
RN, PhD, FAAN**

**Sally Ambler Hutchinson,
RN, PhD, FAAN**

Delmar Publishers
I(T)P An International Thomson Publishing Company

Albany • Bonn • Boston • Cincinnati • Detroit • London • Madrid • Melbourne
Mexico City • New York • Pacific Grove • Paris • San Francisco • Singapore
Tokyo • Toronto • Washington

NOTICE TO THE READER

Cover Design: Timothy J. Conners

Delmar staff:

Publisher: Diane McOscar
Acquisitions Editor: Patricia E. Casey
Production Coordinator: Sandra F. Woods
Art and Design Coordinator: Timothy J. Conners
Editorial Assistant: Tonjia Herman

Copyright © 1996 by Delmar Publishers Inc.
a division of International Thomson Publishing Inc.
The ITP logo is a trademark under license.

Printed in the United States of America

For more information, contact:

Delmar Publishers
3 Columbia Circle, Box 15015
Albany, New York 12212-5015

International
Thomson Publishing Europe
Berkshire House 168-173
High Holborn
London, WC1V 7AA
England

Thomas Nelson Australia
102 Dodds Street
South Melbourne, 3205
Victoria, Australia

Nelson Canada
1120 Birchmont Road
Scarborough, Ontario
Canada, M1K 5G4

International Thomson Editores
Campos Eliseos 385, Piso 7
Col Polanco
11560 Mexico D F Mexico

International
Thomson Publishing GmbH
Königswinterer Strasse 418
53227 Bonn
Germany

International
Thomson Publishing Asia
221 Henderson Road
#05-10 Henderson Building
Singapore 0315

International
Thomson Publishing—Japan
Hirakawacho Kyowa Building, 3F
2-2-1 Hirakawacho
Chiyoda-ku, Tokyo 102
Japan

1 2 3 4 5 6 7 8 9 10 XXX 01 00 99 98 97 96 95

Library of Congress Cataloging-in-Publication Data

Wilson, Holly Skodol.
  The Consumer's guide to nursing research : exercises, learning activities, tools, and resources / by Holly Skodol Wilson, Sally Ambler Hutchinson.
    p.   cm.
  Includes bibliographical references and index.
  ISBN 0-8273-6264-1
    1. Nursing—Research. 2. Nursing—Research—Problems, exercises, etc. I. Hutchinson, Sally A. II. Title.
RT81.5.W53 1996   95-34323
610.73′072—dc20   CIP

TABLE OF CONTENTS

PART 4 _Conducting Nursing Research_ . . . . _159_

Exercises:

Preface

WHY READ THIS BOOK?

Nursing research is empowering every nurse's clinical practice. *Our ability to document nursing's contributions is critical to survival in an era of health care "reform," cost containment and general "downsizing" of nursing personnell. Research on patient outcomes related to nursing care has become every nurse's business and responsibility.* Findings from nursing studies are transforming patient care and replacing tradition, authority, and trial and error as the sources of our knowledge base. This consumer's guide book presents in one clear, interesting, accessible and practical form exercises, learning activities, tools and resources for *understanding and applying* research in your everyday clinical work. It offers thoughtfully selected information and examples relevant to becoming an informed consumer of and participant in nursing research. The development of scientific knowledge as the foundation for quality nursing care has been designated as the responsibility of <u>all</u> nurses regardless of educational preparation. Building a scientific basis for practice requires a variety of investigative skills and competencies if we are to tease out the knowledge embedded in our clinical work. *The Consumer's Guide to Nursing Research* offers all nursing students and practicing nurses a creative, engaging, action-oriented approach for making the research process as familiar and useful as the nursing process in your patient care. This book demonstrates that like Wagner's music, nursing research is better than it sounds.

CONTENTS

The rich array of topics covered in this guide book are well reflected in the detailed Table of Contents. They include all the areas you would expect to learn about as a beginning student of nursing research. They are, however, presented in a more palatable, informal and interactional style than you would find in most introductory research methods books. Students have the opportunity to learn research terms, concepts, methods and processes using engaging, action-oriented exercises, activities, tools and resources. Each of the guide book parts begins with a succinct informative introduction and contains resources, readings and references that are interesting and relevant to expanding research know-how.

They are all coded, using logos for:

☞ . . . . teacher assistance needed

📖 . . . . additional library time/resources

🔆 . . . . difficulty or intensity

⏱ . . . . time-intensive.

An appendix includes answers to exercises. End papers present commonly used statistical symbols. Commonly used statistical tables also appear in an appendix. Finally, a glossary of key terms identified by boldface type throughout the book and an index appear at the end. Unlike many other student workbooks and manuals, *The Consumer's Guide to Nursing Research* presents a format that fosters active learning through a creative approach. Activities, exercises, tools and resources are grouped into parts that each begin with a narrative of essential information helpful in completing the activity or exercise. All examples are drawn from contemporary nursing research literature. Features of particular interest include:

• A values clarification exercise for assessing attitudes toward nursing research

• Vocabulary games for learning research terminology

• Structured critique exercises for studies that use different designs

• A guide for transforming clinical questions into researchable problems

• A list of good writing rules.

AUDIENCE

The Consumer's Guide to Nursing Research is written for entry level nursing students including those enrolled in Diploma, Associate and Baccalaureate degree programs. It can be used whether research is integrated in the curriculum or taught as a separate class or course. It is also a valuable resource for practicing nurses who have the opportunity to participate in research studies, implement research findings or attend in-service, staff development programs focused on nursing research. Nurses returning to graduate school would benefit from using this book as a review—especially if a few years have passed since their undergraduate days. This is a book for all students and clinicians who appreciate the need for advancing nursing research and as intelligent consumers and critics want a highly practical concise resource to guide their involvement. In addition to using the book as a student supplement to a research text, it also can stand alone because part introductions, back of the book answers, utilization logos and the glossary create a self-contained learning package. Faculty who are teaching introductory research classes or courses or who simply choose to teach the scientific basis of all nursing can also rely on this guide book as a source of interactional exercises and activities for classroom and post-conference clinical discussion. We urge users to validate, refine, and further develop these tools based on experience with them and to correspond with us about their findings because these tools have not yet been scientifically validated.

RELATIONSHIP TO THE *CORE INTRODUCTORY NURSING TEXTBOOK SERIES (CINTS)*

While not in and of itself a cornerstone of the Core Introductory Nursing Textbook Series (CINTS), *The Consumer's Guide to Nursing Research* is a valuable adjunct. It shares the commitment to values of "The Curriculum Revolution" that shift from delivering content to students to empowering students as critical thinkers. This book invites students to become full partners in nursing's research enterprise.

ACKNOWLEDGMENTS

The authors wish to acknowledge the assistance of Denise Figueroa, BSN in library research for this book.

We wish also to express our gratitude to the nurses and nursing students who realize that in this era of health care cost-containment and cut-backs, learning about nursing research has become every nurse's business and essential to our profession's empowerment.

In addition, specific thanks go to this book's reviewers for their insight, wisdom and helpful suggestions.

- Kathleen A. De Lorenzo PhD, RN, CS
  University of Central Arkansas
  Conway, Arkansas

- Mary Finnick gnsh, EdD, RN
  University at Buffalo State University of New York
  Buffalo, New York

- Diana D. Hankes, RN, PhD, CS
  Carroll College
  Columbia College of Nursing
  Milwaukee, Wisconsin

Last but not least, we express our appreciation to Patricia Casey, our sponsoring editor at Delmar for believing in the value of this Guidebook and for rallying as its advocate during the stormy course of coming to print.

To our friendship
(1960 - forever)
HSW & SAH
1996

PART 1

Competence in Nursing Research: Professional Empowerment

✢ Ways of Knowing

A sexually active 41-year-old advertising executive from Boston asks you if it is safe to continue using an intrauterine device (IUD) as her method of birth control. An affluent mother in a California suburb confides that she begins drinking as soon as her teenage children leave for school. She is depressed but ashamed to admit it because all the other women she knows have "gotten it all altogether." You observe a few drops of bright red blood on a neonate in a neonatal intensive care unit (NICU). Is it just oozing, or is the infant's arterial line no longer patent? A homeless diabetic patient is brought into an urban emergency room in a comatose state. How do you decide if the patient suffers from insulin shock or is in a diabetic coma?

Regardless of the degree of sophistication that educated individuals bring to the nursing profession, we continue to rely on diverse "ways of knowing" when responding to important and difficult clinical questions such as those just described:

- Trial and error combined with common sense
- Authority and tradition following stated rules and procedure books
- Inspiration and intuition
- Logical reasoning
- Scientific research

The scientific approach to research is the focus of this **Consumer's Guidebook.**

What is the Scientific Approach?

The scientific approach to research is a process of learning about the truth. It is:

- Not dogmatic and mechanical
- Not just a process of proof
- Not just knowledge of irrefutable facts devoid of interpretation
- Not esoteric, incomprehensible, and unrelated to real-world problems of clinical practice.

The **scientific approach** is a *process by which observable, verifiable data are systematically collected from the world we know through our senses to describe, explain, and/or predict events*. The scientific approach to knowing has two characteristics that the other approaches do not: (1) self-correction or objectivity, and (2) the use of sensory, or *empirical, data*.

A system of checks is built into the investigation process so that if a scientist finds a particular explanation is supported, that scientist will also test alternative explanations. This testing in turn must be open to the criticism of others. Furthermore, the appeal to empirical data that characterizes the scientific method is done in a systematic way according to canons or a consensus of rules or conventions. The intentions of scientific inquiry are: (1) to develop explanations called theories and (2) to find solutions to existing practical problems.

Nursing Research Priorities

Some authors make a distinction between what is called *nursing research* (that is, research into the process of care and the clinical problems encountered in the practice of nursing) and *research in nursing* (the broader study of people and the nursing profession, including historic, ethical, and political studies). Predictions for nursing research are that it will continue to emphasize studies of the interaction of physiologic and psychosocial mechanisms in human experiences of stress and coping, evaluations of nursing interventions, the transfer of research findings into textbooks and practice, a focus on the underserved and high-risk groups such as the elderly, the chronically mentally ill, and minorities, and the creation of a body of scientific nursing knowledge. You as a student or clinician of today will be directly involved in its conduct and application.

Understanding Research Articles

An essential skill for you as intelligent consumer, evaluator, and applier of research findings to your practice is mastering the fine art of active reading. *The amount of what you comprehend in a report of research findings often depends on the amount of active thinking you put into the process of reading.*

Techniques for Active Reading

Active reading involves you in a process of actively questioning the material you read. Some devices that can help you accomplish this fruitfully include the following:

1. Quickly read the title page, preface, or abstract to get an idea of the topic of the article or book and categorize it in your mind. Is it really a report of findings, or is it a "dwell and tell" anecdotal account of somebody's isolated experience?
2. Study the table of contents or headings in the piece to get a sense of its structure. This should alert you in advance of what to expect.
3. Read any boldface excerpts or boxed summaries to ascertain the article's main point or ideas.
4. Leaf through the whole piece, dipping in here and there for a paragraph.

5. Find the important and unfamiliar words and determine their meanings. Use resources like this book's glossary or a good nursing dictionary.
6. Highlight key points or conclusions by underlining or putting stars or asterisks in the margin.
7. Construct the article's basic logic or premises, and determine what results have been found or what conclusions have been reached.
8. Be able to say with certainty that you understand what you've read before you criticize it or ask "What of it?"
9. Compare what you read in one source with what you've read cumulatively on a topic.

Finding Research Literature

Before reports of research findings can be evaluated for usefulness to your practice, you must be able to locate them. There are currently many nursing journals with an editorial policy that stresses science and research: *Nursing Research, Advances in Nursing Science, Journal of Research in Nursing and Health,* and the *Western Journal of Nursing Research* are among the most well-known. Research studies also are sometimes published in general nursing journals like the *American Journal of Nursing* and in specialty journals like *Heart and Lung.* The Mosby Year Books journal entitled *Capsules and Comments,* published quarterly, abstracts studies and provides expert comments about their relevance. Most major texts also include thoughtfully selected research notes. The *Cumulative Index to Nursing and Allied Health Literature,* the *International Nursing Index,* the *Cumulative Medical Index,* and computerized literature searches such as MEDLINE and MEDLARS are resources for locating articles on a topic that is relevant to your work.

✛ Identifying Researchable Problems: An Investigative Role for All Nurses

Over a decade ago a special Commission on Nursing Research appointed by the American Nurses' Association (ANA) published an official statement emphasizing that building a scientific base for clinical practice is the most important priority for nursing research. Furthermore, they agreed that if such a goal is to be reached, all nurses, including those prepared in diploma and associate degree programs, have important roles: (1) in becoming aware of the value of research for improving nursing practice, (2) assisting in the collection of data in clinical situations, and (3) especially in identifying research questions that are important to advancing knowledge about patient care and the outcome of nursing interventions or nursing systems.

The exercises in Part I, which focus on research problems, will provide strategies for considering sources of research questions, ways of differentiating between clinical problems that can be studied using the scientific method and those that cannot, and criteria for recognizing the different kinds of research problems that serve as the starting point for studies that you may read. Knowing the characteristics of a good research question will help you formulate study problems on your own and judge whether the research you read is relevant to clinical problems in your practice. An intelligent consumer of research studies must begin by understanding exactly what question the research is attempting to answer.

✤ Bridging the Research–Practice Gap

Leaders in nursing emphasize the need for a bridge between the research–practice gap. This involves a two-way process of making nursing practice a more frequent focus for research and of increasing the application of research findings to practice. Most authorities agree that applying research to practice would be a lot easier if:

- The scientific community were closer to bringing some sense of order to the growing body of nursing research
- All nursing students were better prepared to find, read, and understand nursing research
- Service organizations were structured to foster such applications

Most onlookers seem to characterize nursing research as discrete, nonaggregated studies of isolated empirical phenomena for which the underlying theory is not known or not yet well-defined.

Despite the impressive past progress in the advancement of nursing science and research, problems still arise when the means for translating nursing research findings into practice decisions are examined. Present barriers to the advancement of nursing research include the following:

1. Nursing has not yet systematically reviewed and collected its important research reports.
2. Few examples of replicating prior scientific work can be found in nursing literature and practice.
3. Researchers and clinicians don't communicate and interact about findings that have implications for practice.

These barriers, however, have not obstructed all progress. In less than 30 years, nursing research has shifted from the study of the profession itself (studies of supply distribution, job satisfaction, job turnover, and education) to the study of phenomena with which nursing is concerned: the problems and processes of nursing care.

Values Clarification—Where Do You Stand in Relation to Nursing Research?

The following values clarification exercise is designed to help you get in touch with where you stand on the issue of your involvement in nursing research.

Directions

The following box or graph is a **semantic differential** designed for you to rank your feelings about nursing research. Put a check in the box in each row that best reflects the value of your feelings.

How I Feel About Nursing Research

Interested								Bored
Confident								Afraid
Pleasant								Unpleasant
Good								Bad
Warm								Cold
Invigorated								Tired
Curious								Disinterested
Adequate								Inadequate
Comfortable								Uncomfortable
Inspired								Turned off

Discussion Guidelines

Look at where you put your checks. Note the extremes at the far left or right and those in the middle, and determine if your feelings about research are predominantly negative or positive and whether they are strongly or mildly so. Think about *why* you feel the way you do. Respond to the following questions in your discussion.

1. What has influenced your feelings?
2. What could you do to alter your feelings if they are negative?

How Nurses Approach and "Know" About Clinical Problems

Nurses approach clinical problems with diverse ways of knowing, including: (a) trial and error and common sense, (b) authority and tradition, (c) inspiration and intuition and, (d) logical reasoning or science. Some examples of the application of these ways of knowing are reflected in the clinical situations that follow.

Directions

Indicate by letter listed above which of the ways of knowing apply in the following situations:

_____ 1. Mr. Jones was recently diagnosed as having cancer of the lung. In spite of a poor prognosis indicating that he would die within a few months, he talked happily about his plans to travel around the world with his wife and start a new business, which was a life long dream. The nurse recognized he was in the initial stage of denial, according to Kübler-Ross' theory of dying, and permitted him to discuss his dreams.

_____ 2. Mrs. Smith was scheduled to have an abortion following an amniocentesis that identified multiple congenital defects of the fetus. Mrs. Smith asked the nurse's opinion on abortion. The nurse replied that she felt amniocentesis was not always accurate, and she personally would not have an abortion.

_____ 3. Mrs. Castro, from Colombia, South America, was hospitalized for renal failure. Her four children and their spouses, her parents, her husband, and sisters came to the hospital daily and stayed for several hours, requesting to participate in Mrs. Castro's care. Because this was against policy, the nurse in charge refused their admittance and help, resulting in anger and frustration for everyone involved.

_____ 4. A young man was brought into the emergency room after taking an indeterminant amount of Valium. His vital signs were stable, and he was alert and oriented. The nurse called the attending physician and recommended the patient be discharged, since he seemed fine and she had never before seen Valium hurt anyone. She told his family to bring him back to the emergency room if any problems developed.

_____ 5. Nurse X was concerned about Janet, a 15-year-old girl, admitted to the psychiatric ward for depression. Janet was disappearing into the bathroom after every meal and subsequently losing weight rapidly. Nurse X suspected she was vomiting her meals (a condition known as bulimia), so she asked two other nurses on the other shifts to subtly watch Janet immediately after eating and report their observations to her.

_____ 6. A patient who had undergone cardiac bypass surgery was afraid to have sexual intercourse. The nurse believed that sexual intercourse would be similar to moderate exercise, which was allowed, and told the patient to resume sexual activity without worrying. In the nurse's experience, no cardiac patient had ever died from sexual intercourse.

_____ 7. Nurse A noticed Nurse B lingering near the medicine cabinet. Nurse B disappeared into the bathroom and appeared a few minutes later with a glazed look in her eyes and bandages on the back of her hands. Nurse A knew stealing and using drugs was a violation of the nurse practice act so she reported Nurse B to the head nurse.

_____ 8. Mr. X was dying. His nurse, a person with strong religious beliefs, called a chaplain. The patient refused to see the chaplain, saying that his spiritual beliefs were personal and that he did not want any outsiders to see him. Regardless of Mr. X's objections, the nurse sent the chaplain in anyway.

Answers to be found at the back of the book.

Discussion Guidelines

Think about each of the preceding situations, and decide on the steps you would take to solve each dilemma using logical scientific reasoning. Discuss your conclusions with a fellow student or a small group in your research seminar.

Active Reading to Increase Clinical Knowledge

As a professional nurse, you will want to read on a variety of topics related to your clinical interests. Articles on theory, research, and practice will be part of your repertoire. Acquiring active reading skills requires your proficiency in the four levels of reading:

1. Elementary reading • initial or rudimentary reading
2. Systematic skimming • prereading
3. Analytic reading • asking questions of what you are reading:
   a. What is the book or journal article about as a whole? (You search for the fundamental theme.)
   b. What is being said in detail and how? (You search for the main ideas, assertions, and arguments.)
   c. Is the book or article true in whole or part?
   d. What is the significance of what you have read?
4. Comparative reading • relating what you have read to the larger body of knowledge on the same subject.

Assuming you are already proficient at elementary reading and systematic skimming, do the following exercise to improve your skills of analytic reading.

Directions

Pick one journal article or book that relates to a clinical area of interest to you or in which you are presently working. Read the article or book and respond to the questions for analytic reading. Write your answers down, returning to the work as often as you must until you feel you really do understand it.

Discussion Guidelines

To improve your proficiency in comparative reading, write a few paragraphs about what you have just read and its relationship to what you have previously read on the same subject. Or, if you haven't read on the same subject, look up additional related articles in the *Cumulative Nursing Index*. Then ask yourself the following questions regarding the material you have read.

1. Is there agreement on the topic or some controversy?
2. Where does the controversy lie?
3. Are there suggestions for additional studies?

As you repeat this process over and over, you will find yourself thinking more as you read, resulting in increased comprehension and a sense of relatedness.

Peer Collaboration in Implementation of Nursing Research

Implementation of nursing research in a clinical setting requires active participation by many nurses. Nurses from Associate (AD), Bachelor of Science (BS), and Master degree (MS) programs all have a role.

Directions

Read one of the research articles listed in the references that follow. Divide your group of students or colleagues into three sections and have each section discuss a plan to answer one of the following questions:

1. If the research is implemented, what should be the role of nurses with Associate degrees?
2. The role of nurses with Bachelor of Science degrees?
3. The role of nurses with Masters degrees?

Relate the nurses' roles specifically to the requirements for implementing the research in practice.

Discussion Guidelines

After 30 minutes of discussion, the three sections should meet together as one group; a spokesperson from each section should share their plan with the larger group. The following questions can be used as a discussion guide:

1. Can you clearly articulate the role of nurses from each educational level?
2. What are the specific duties required by the implementation of the particular research project that will be performed by nurses from each level?

References

Brown, S. A. (1992). Meta-Analysis of diabetes patient education research: Variations in intervention effects across studies. *Research in Nursing and Health, 15*(16), 409–419.

Sideranko, S., Quinn, A., Burns, K., & Froman, R. D. (1992). Effects of position and mattress overlay on sacral and heel pressures in a clinical population. *Research in Nursing and Health, 15*(4), 245–251.

Tesler, M. D., Savadra, L., Holzemer, W., Wilkie, D. J., Ward, J. A., & Paul, S. M. (1991). The word-graphic rating scale as a measure of children's and adolescents' pain intensity. *Research in Nursing and Health, 14*(15), 361–371.

Topf, M. (1992). Effects of personal control over hospital noise on sleep. *Research in Nursing and Health, 15*(1), 19–28.

Dreaming Up a Good Clinical Study

Good clinical studies have the following characteristics in common (Fuller, 1982):

1. They study a problem that occurs frequently in a definable population of patients.
2. The standard way of managing the problem is unsatisfactory.
3. Some index of the problem can be measured.
4. The proposed solution alters patient care.

Directions

Think about your clinical experiences in nursing, and write a plan for research that meets the characteristics just given. Your plan should address all four characteristics.

Discussion Guidelines

Meet with a group of fellow students or colleagues, and take turns presenting ideas for a clinical study. The following questions should help you in your discussion.

1. Is the problem frequently occurring?
2. Is the present way of managing the problem unsatisfactory? Why?
3. Can the problem be measured by a specific index? How?
4. Will the solution alter patient care? How?
5. What are some suggestions for improving on the study?

Reference

Fuller, E. (1982). Selecting a clinical nursing problem for research. *Image: Journal of Nursing Scholarship*, June, *14*, 60–61.

Sources of Research Problems

Personal life experience, patterns, or trends in clinical practice, somebody else's completed research reports, and your intellectual and scientific interests are all valid sources of research problems in nursing. Recognition of these sources is one way to make you aware of potential research problems.

Directions

The sources of research problems just mentioned are listed at the left. Think about each source, and write an example in the right column from your own personal or nursing experience.

Sources of Research Problems	Example Research Problems
1. Experience a. Wishes and desires	1.
b. Complaints	
c. Questions	

2. Patterns or trends   2.

3. Completed research (i.e.,   3.
    reported research, case studies,
    clinical descriptions)

4. Your intellectual and scientific   4
    interests

Discussion Guidelines

Discuss your examples with your colleagues or fellow students. If you had all the time in the world and access to unlimited resources, which of your examples would you choose to study? Why?

Researchable and Nonresearchable Questions

If you are going to participate in research yourself, or evaluate the usefulness of research that you read, you must be able to distinguish between a question that is researchable and a question that is nonresearchable. A researchable problem is one that can be investigated using the process of **scientific inquiry**. Two major types of nonresearchable questions are (1) value, or "should," questions and (2) "yes" or "no" questions.

Directions

Read the following questions, and indicate what are researchable (R) or nonresearchable (NR) in the spaces provided to the left. Change all the questions you believe to be nonresearchable into researchable questions.

_____ 1. Is ice water harmful to patients with myocardial infarctions?

_____ 2. Should all diabetics learn to give themselves insulin?

_____ 3. Which of two staff patterns is most effective in increasing the recovery rate (decreasing hospital stay) of open-heart patients?

_____ 4. Should nurses in psychiatric units wear white uniforms?

_____ 5. Do self-hypnosis techniques help patients with chronic pain?

_____ 6. What are the attitudes of labor and delivery nurses toward nurse midwives?

_____ 7. What should be the role of the clinical specialist (RN with a Master degree)?

_____ 8. Do dying children have spiritual needs?

_____ 9. What are the patients' perceptions of the most preferred methods of control (seclusion alone, restraints with seclusion, or restraints alone) for combative psychotic patients?

_____10. Do nurses with Associate degrees meet the social–psychological needs of patients?

_____11. Should the Baylor Plan be instituted at all hospitals?

_____12. Which of the two types of pulmonary toilet is most effective with patients with cardiopulmonary disease?

Discussion Guidelines

Discuss with your colleagues or fellow students the nonresearchable questions you rewrote to be researchable.

1. Are they no longer value, or "should" questions?
2. Are they no longer questions that can be answered with a simple "yes" or "no?"

Answers to be found at the back of the book.

8

Types of Research Questions

An awareness of the types of research questions helps you think about your practice in terms of research. You will view occurrences in your practice differently, and you will begin to think about possible research questions.

Directions

Types of researchable questions are listed in the left column. In the right column, write an example of each type from your practice or personal experience.

Types   Example

Why are things this way?

What would happen if . . . ?

Which approach would work better?

Who might benefit from this?

Discussion Guidelines

Discuss your examples with your colleagues or fellow students. Are all your examples researchable? If not, why not?

9

Learning to Apply Research Studies to Guide Nursing Practice

Ideally, nursing research and research adapted from other disciplines guide practice decisions and, thus, ultimately affect patient care. This exercise is designed to help you assess studies from the nursing literature and decide if you and your co-workers or fellow students would want to apply the study findings to your nursing practice.

Directions

Read one or more of the articles in the reference list that is related to your work.

Discussion Guidelines

Discuss the following questions with a group of colleagues or fellow students.

1. Does application of the study findings in the particular practice setting make sense to you? Are they useful? Are they clear?
2. How would patient care differ if you implemented any of the knowledge from these studies in your unit? Or to your clinical laboratory experience?
3. Do you foresee any problems connected with implementing knowledge generated in these studies? (This includes patient care, nursing problems, administrative, etc.)
4. What would be the cost/benefit ratio of implementing this research knowledge?

References

Fetter, M., & Lowery, B. (1992). Psychiatric rehospitalization of the severely mentally ill: Patient and staff perspectives. *Nursing Research, 41*(5), 301–305.

Jemmott, L., & Jemmott, J. (1992). Increasing condom-use intentions among sexually active black adolescent women. *Nursing Research, 41*(5), 273–279.

Kirkevold, M. (1993). Toward a practice theory of caring for patients with chronic skin disease. *Scholarly Inquiry for Nursing Practice: An International Journal, 7*(1), 37–52.

Lindenberg, C., Gendrop, S., & Reiskin, H. (1993). Empirical evidence for the social stress model of substance abuse. *Research in Nursing and Health, 16*(5), 351–362.

Murphy, S. (1993). Coping strategies of abstainers from alcohol up to three years post-treatment. *Image, 25*(1), 29–35.

O'Brien, B., & Pearson, A. (1993). Unwritten knowledge in nursing: Consider the spoken as well as the written word. *Scholarly Inquiry for Nursing Practice: An International Journal, 7*(2), 111–124.

PART   2

History, Ethics and Philosophy of Nursing Research

✤   The History of Nursing Research

Many authorities believe that nursing research dates back to 1853–1856 when Florence Nightingale recorded detailed observations about the impact of nursing care during the Crimean War, thus fostering the idea that nursing practice should be based on disciplined inquiry. It was not until 1923 and the publication of The Goldmark Report reporting on a comprehensive study of nursing education sponsored by the Committee for the Study of Nursing Education and funded by the Rockefeller Foundation that advanced educational preparation was deemed essential for teachers, administrators, and public health nurses. Yale University's School of Nursing was established that same year with The Vanderbilt University and Western Reserve University Schools of Nursing soon to follow. The real pioneers had been Teachers' College, Columbia (1899) and the University of Minnesota (1910)—the first schools to emphasize higher education for nurses. By 1948, another important report was published. The Brown Report recommended studies of in-service education, nursing functions, nursing teams, nurse-patient relationships, hospital environments, and the economic security of nurses. Soon thereafter in 1952, *Nursing Research*, the first official journal for reporting studies related to nursing and health was established to offer nurse investigators a means for communicating the results of their research. A year later The Institute of Research and Service in Nursing Education was founded at Columbia University under the directorship of Dr. Helen Bunge. It became the first formal structure within a university for conducting nursing studies. By 1955 The American Nurses' Foundation was established by ANA to serve as a receiver, administrator, and donor of grants for research in nursing. That same year the nursing research grants and fellowship program of the Division of Nursing of the then U.S. Public Health Service began awarding grants for research into causes, diagnosis, treatment, and control of physical, and mental diseases. By 1957 The Department of Nursing in The Walter Reed Army Institute of Research was established alongside medicine and dentistry to develop a core of nurse practitioner-researchers. Six years later in 1963, Lydia Hall conducted a classic study of care of chronically ill patients at the Loeb Rehabilitation Center in New York and, as an example of research on patient care, it influenced the emergence of conceptual frameworks to define the nature of nursing practice. Research on social/psychological aspects of health and illness was initiated in 1966 by a team of nurse researchers collaborating with sociologists Glaser and Strauss at the University of California School of Nursing, and qualitative sociological methods called "The Discovery of Grounded Theory" began to appear in nursing studies. In 1968 The Mugar Library at Boston University established the first nursing archive and throughout the subsequent decade numerous refereed research journals for nursing were published offering nurse researchers more opportunities for communicating their study findings to the growing community of nurse scientists. By 1983 The American Nurses' Association had created the First Center for Nursing Research and by 1986 The National Center for Nursing Research (NCNR) was established as part of the National Institutes of Health (NIH) by congressional mandate. Finally, in 1993 the NCNR became a full-fledged Institute of the NIH. The National Institute for Nursing Research (NINR) has placed nursing research in the mainstream of scientific investigation focused on our nation's health.

✤ Research Ethics

Ethics is a branch of philosophy concerned with two basic questions: (1) "What is right or good?" and (2) "What should I do?" Because nursing research tends to focus on humans it is a major nursing responsibility to be aware of a person's right to **informed consent** and that an appropriate *balance exists between the risks and potential benefits of participating in the study.*

Characteristics of Ethical Research

Ethical research includes protecting the rights of human subjects, but also encompasses a broader list of characteristics. Most of these characteristics are reflected in a document entitled the American Nurses' Association's Human Rights Guidelines for Nursing in Clinical and Other Research and are based on historic efforts such as the Nuremberg Code, the Declaration of Helsinki, and United States federal regulations, which set standards governing human research.

The Institutional Review Board

Although it is the responsibility of all investigators to examine their own studies with good conscience and complete candor, federal regulations require that institutions, including universities, hospitals, nursing homes, and health agencies, establish review committees on human research, called **Institutional Review Boards (IRBs)**. Most review boards have instructions for investigators that include steps to be taken to receive approval, forms for human-subjects protocols, guidelines for writing a standard consent form, and criteria for qualifying for an expedited rather than full committee review. Institutional review boards make final decisions on all federally funded research protocols involving human subjects. Their duty is to protect subjects from undue risk and deprivation of personal rights and dignity. This protection is achieved by reviewing a study's protocol to ensure that it meets the major requirements of ethical research and that the consent process, as reflected in the consent form, promotes the free self-determination of potential subjects.

Vulnerable Subjects

You can expect a board reviewing a nursing study to exercise special care if the research involves subjects with diminished capacity to give free and informed consent. Minors, prisoners, unconscious persons, the mentally retarded, students, and employees must be aware that their care, job, or status is in no way dependent on serving as research subjects. A formal consent document is one way of putting the agreement between the investigator and the subjects into written form; letters of agreement, information sheets, or verbal consent are alternatives. The main principle is that *it is the scientist's responsibility to tell a reasonable person in language that he or she can understand the information he or she would wish to know in order to make an informed decision.*

✜ The Nurse's Role

Advocates for research subjects, your own conscience, and impartial review committees are methods of safeguarding the rights of human research subjects. Nurses who are investigators themselves or who assist in the research of others are in a key position to assert and maintain the protective values to which our profession is committed. A study design that deprived one group of patients of relaxation techniques for labor pain or preoperative teaching, for example, would be unethical unless provisions were made for alternatively effective care.

The exercises and activities that follow in Part 2 give you an opportunity to apply this information and these ideas.

Dominant Philosophies of Science Applied in Nursing Research

Despite the commonly accepted characteristics and intentions of the scientific approach, scientists themselves can differ in their views of this approach. To capture the subtle diversity here and its meaning for the way research studies are designed, the dominant perspectives on the philosophy of science must be considered.

Two schools of thought, sometimes called intellectual traditions, are the basis for most nursing research. The first is called the **positivist tradition**, and the second, the **naturalistic/interpretive, tradition.** The positivists subscribe to the following opinions about nursing science:

1. Nurse scientists can and do attain *objective* knowledge of both the physical and social worlds.
2. The logic of inquiry and procedure for conducting research should be the same whether one is studying plants or people.
3. Social order in the universe is relatively mechanistic.
4. Objectivity in research can be obtained in setting forth a highly controlled and preplanned research design.

The nonpositivist, or naturalistic/interpretive advocates subscribe to a different set of beliefs with implications for discovering the truth, including:

1. Fundamental differences exist between the natural or physical sciences and the psychosocial sciences, and different research methods are required for each.
2. Research studies that consider the whole person, as do nursing studies, must take into account the subjective aspects of human experience.
3. There is no objective reality waiting to be measured.
4. If nurse scientists are to comprehend people, they must understand each person's definition of his or her own reality.
5. Human order and patterns are constantly in a state of becoming, and scientists therefore cannot presume to impose rigid pre-established categories on phenomena without forcing the fit.

The consequences of adhering to one or the other of these major scientific philosophies is that positivists advocate research methods governed by the rules of testing **hypotheses** and verifying **theory** borrowed from hard sciences like physics. Conversely, naturalistic/interpretive advocates in the traditions of anthropology and sociology emphasize first-hand knowledge under natural conditions, using whatever observational strategies are meaningful and useful.

Historic Landmarks in Nursing Research

General understanding of the history of nursing research helps put the present in perspective. The following matching exercise lists historic events and their outcomes.

Directions

Reread the Introduction to this part and match the outcome provided in the column on the right with the event described in the left column. Place the corresponding number from the outcome column in the space provided at the left.

Events

_____ 1. In 1923, the Goldmark Report, a comprehensive study of nursing education, was published.

_____ 2. In 1853–1856, Florence Nightingale recorded detailed observations about the impact of nursing care during the Crimean War.

_____ 3. In 1948, the Brown report was published.

_____ 4. In 1952, *Nursing Research*, the first nursing research journal, was published.

_____ 5. In 1953, the first Institute of Research and Service in Nursing Education was established at Columbia University.

_____ 6. In 1955, the ANA established the American Nurses' Foundation.

_____ 7. In 1955, the nursing research grants and fellowship program of the Division of Nursing of the U.S. Public Health Service was established.

_____ 8. In 1957, the Department of Nursing in the Walter Reed Army Institute of Research was established.

Outcomes

1. Serves as a receiver and administrator of grants and as a donor of grants for research in nursing.

2. Generated the idea that nursing practice should be based on disciplined inquiry.

3. The first in a group of scientific journals to provide nurse investigators with means for communicating results of their research.

4. a. Recommended many studies of nursing, nursing education, nursing teams, nurse–patient relationships, hospital environments, and so on.
   b. Began the National Accrediting Service, which aimed to establish a sound method of accrediting nursing education programs.

5. Hoped to develop a core of nurse practitioners–researchers and to accomplish patient-care research paralleling research done by physicians and dentists.

6. First formal structure within a university conducting nursing studies.

7. a. Recommended that advanced educational preparation was essential for teachers, administrators, and public health nurses.

_____ 9. In 1963, the Surgeon General's Consultant Group on Nursing issued a report on its study of the nursing situation.

_____10. In 1963, Lydia Hall conducted a classic study of care for the chronically ill patients at the Loeb Rehabilitation Center in New York.

_____11. In 1966, nurse researchers and sociologists Glaser and Strauss collaborated on death and dying studies.

_____12. In 1968, the Mugar Library at Boston University established a nursing archive.

_____13. In 1970, the Lysaught Report (the National Commission for the Study of Nursing and Nursing Education) was published.

_____14. In 1976, Carnegie reported on the steady increase in the number of clinical investigations published in *Nursing Research*.

_____15. In 1976, the ANA Commission on Research recommended that preparation for nursing research begin at the undergraduate level.

_____16. From 1968 to the present, the Western Interstate Commission for Higher Education in Nursing (WICHEN) compiled data-collection instruments for practice and education, sponsored Communicating Nursing Research Conferences and workshops on conducting and applying research findings in practice.

b. Encouraged the practice of hiring registered nurses for hospital care to free nursing students to study.

c. Yale University's School of Nursing was established to prepare scientific leaders in nursing with University degrees. Vanderbilt (1925) and Western Reserve (1923) Schools of Nursing followed Teachers' College (1899) and University of Minnesota (1910), the first universities to emphasize the higher education of nurses.

8. Authorized grant award programs for research on cause, diagnosis, treatment, control, and prevention of physical and mental disease.

9. Courses and integrated objectives requiring some level of research competence appeared in nursing curricula.

10. Aimed to foster nursing research and bring together a significant collection on the topic.

11. Recommended a substantial increase in federal support for research in nursing and the training of nurse researchers.

12. Sociological methods and concepts began to appear in the repertoire of nurse researchers.

13. The value of clinical or practice-related research was becoming dominant over studies of nurses themselves or education and administration studies.

14. Increased the visibility of nursing's growing involvement in research and methodological sophistication.

15. Examples of research on patient care began to influence the emergence of conceptual frameworks to define the nature of nursing practice.

_____17. In the 1970s, a number of research journals for nursing were established including *Advances in Nursing Science, Research in Nursing and Health,* and *The Western Journal of Nursing Research.*

_____18. In 1986, The National Center for Nursing Research (NCNR) was established as part of the National Institute of Health (NIH) by congressional mandate.

_____19. In 1986, the National Nursing Research Agenda (NNRA) was created.

_____20. In 1993, the National Institute of Nursing Research (NINR) was created.

16. Agreed that research in both nursing education and practice be funded.

17. Offered nurse researchers vehicles through which to communicate their study findings to a growing community of nurse scientists.

18. Emphasizing treatment effectiveness or "outcome research," this agency is funded for studies including nursing clinical practice.

19. Placed nursing research in the mainstream of scientific investigation focused on the nation's health, primarily in patient care, promotion of health, prevention of disease, and the mitigation of effects of acute and chronic illness and disabilities.

20. Developed a five-year plan to provide directions for nursing research within the discipline, culminating in a national conference on research priorities held in January 1989.

Answers to be found at the back of the book.

Discussion Guidelines

After completing the matching exercise, discuss the following questions with your colleagues or fellow students.

1. Which event do you feel has been the most significant in influencing nursing today?
2. The National Institute of Nursing Research (NINR) has been signed into law and given a budget. What do you see as the effects of this historic landmark?

The History of Nursing's Use of Research Findings

According to the article "Factors Encouraging and Discouraging the Use of Nursing Research Findings" (Pettengill et al., 1994), "nurses have steadily increased the amount and quality of their research (p. 143)." Yet research findings according to experts are not yet being used in clinical practice.

Directions

After reading the above-mentioned article discuss the topics that follow in a group of colleagues or fellow students.

Discussion Topics

1. What was the purpose of the Pettengill et al. article?
2. What questions guided their research?
3. Describe the study sample and the selection process.
4. What did the authors learn about the factors that encouraged or discouraged use of nursing research findings?
5. Which of them apply to you in your studies or your clinical work at the present time?

Reference

Pettengill, M. M., Gellies, D. A., & Clark, C. C. (1994). Factors encouraging and discouraging the use of nursing research findings. *Image: Journal of Nursing Scholarship*, 26(2), 143–147.

Making Ethical Decisions When You Are Involved in Research

All scientific research has ethical dimensions that must be addressed. As patient advocate, it is the nurse's role to raise ethical questions and to assess the answers to ensure that each study participated in meets ethical requirements. The following vignettes reveal common ethical dilemmas that practicing nurses are likely to confront. Thinking ahead about how to solve potential problems should help mobilize and prepare you when they arise.

Directions

Read the following vignettes, and then respond to the question provided in the Discussion Guidelines.

1. A surgeon, Dr. X, is doing research on how fast certain dyes go through the hepatic circulatory system. During surgery, he tries out three different dyes. You, the operating room nurse, learn through conversation with Dr. X that he does not have Institutional Review Board (IRB) approval for the research. "It's just my own little study," he says. "No reason to go through all that." You are aware that the procedure does increase anesthesia time and could possibly have complications for the patient.

2. You are a nurse on a labor and delivery unit. The chief of Obstetrics and Gynecology asks you to do research with him on Subject X. You like the idea of doing research because you want to learn more, but you are a little worried you might merely become his "gopher." You are afraid of being exploited, yet you are not even sure of all the ways you can be exploited.

3. A cardiologist is doing an approved research study on blood oxygen levels in patients following myocardial infarctions. It would be your responsibility to get informed consent from the patients and to collect the data. You want to help, but you do not fully understand the research or its risks and benefits for the patient. You also recognize that you are not doing nursing research, but are participating in medical research. You think that some nursing research on the patients' responses to the tests would be useful.

4. You are a practicing pediatric nurse who is interested in the effects of patient teaching on adolescents with diabetes. The head nurse has asked you to study the children's responses to having pets on the unit. You do not have time to do both studies.

5. A nursing director assigns you to study her new staffing plan. She is convinced it is working and that "the nurses love it." The results of your study, however, indicate disharmony among the nursing staff and their desire to change the plan. The director chooses to ignore your results, saying the research method led to spurious results.

6. You are studying different techniques and the use of different sites for taping and securing intravenous lines (IVs). You have IRB approval, and you have both a control and an experimental group. Several patients in the experimental group complain of pain at the site and request that the line be put in a different place.

7. You are doing a case study on Mr. X, who is dying of myasthenia gravis. He signed a consent form at the beginning of the study, and you have been interviewing him biweekly over a period of several months. Mr. X is currently very depressed and angry. He tells you he no longer wants to talk to you. He feels like a guinea pig and wants nothing more to do with this research.

8. As a nurse on an intensive care unit, you are aware of numerous ongoing research projects conducted by physicians. You find out that your hospital does have an IRB and that the board is composed of physicians, a pharmacist, and a dentist. You are concerned that there is no representation for nurses. You strongly believe that it is the nurse's role to be the patient advocate and that a nurse has a vital role to play on review boards.

9. You are a participant in a study of nursing care in a psychiatric unit. You become aware of patient abuse—both physical and psychological. For example, one nurse refused to give water to a patient in restraints for the entire shift; you saw nurses and attendants using excess force to restrain patients; you witnessed a nurse laughing at a psychotic patient who thought he was a dog.

10. You have completed your research on nursing in the prison system. You have learned that nurses frequently turn their backs on prisoner abuse by the guards and the police because of their fear that the guards will not protect them from violent prisoners if they report anything amiss. The nursing administration wants you to present your findings.

11. You have given a packet of questionnaires to alcoholics and drug abusers. You have a master list of their names that can be matched with their coded questionnaires. Their therapist, who has given you access to the patients, wants to see the completed questionnaires to identify how each patient answered. He says the information will give him a better idea of how to help them in therapy.

Discussion Guidelines

Discuss the following with a small group of colleagues or fellow students:

1. Identify the problem(s) in each vignette.
2. List the steps you can take to begin to solve the problem(s).
   a. If you believe further information is necessary, write down what you need.
   b. Indicate where you will get this information.
   c. What will you do after you get the information?

Principles of Ethical Research

13

The principles of ethical research include the following:

1. Scientific objectivity
2. Cooperation with duly authorized review groups, agencies, and institutional review boards
3. Integrity in representing the research enterprise
4. Equitability in acknowledging the contributions of others
5. Nobility in the application of processes and procedures to protect the rights of human subjects
6. Truthfulness about a study's purpose, procedures, methods, and findings
7. Impeccability in the use of any privileges that may be associated with the researcher's role
8. Forthrightness about a study's funding sources and sponsorship
9. Illumination of your discipline's body of scientific knowledge through your contribution of publications and presentations of research findings
10. Courage to clarify publicly any distortions that others make of your research findings

Directions

Read the following vignettes. Each vignette is designed to illustrate adherence to or violation of one of the principles of ethical research. After reading each vignette, indicate which principle was adhered to or violated and why you reached this conclusion.

1. A nurse researcher had worked for 3 years on a unit that housed nonviable patients. She was outraged by how the nurses, herself included, categorized these patients and how they consistently avoided certain patients. The nurse designed a qualitative research project in which she planned to observe and interview nurses on her unit to find out "How nurses perceive caring for nonviable patients."
2. A nurse was studying nonprofessional behavior of nurses. Because the subject could be potentially threatening, a social psychologist suggested that the nurse avoid revealing the nature of her research, offering instead only a vague, general description of her study, such as "I'm studying nurses' behavior." The researcher felt uncomfortable with this suggestion and decided to be totally honest and open about her topic, recognizing that some people may withdraw or be unwilling to talk to her.
3. A nurse planned to do a pilot study prior to a more extensive research project on care of decubitus ulcers on bedridden patients. Since it was merely a pilot study and time was limited, the nurse decided not to go through the **Institutional Review Board** (IRB) at this time even though all research involving human subjects is required to do so.
4. In the study of nonprofessional behavior several nurse informants revealed some very personal and potentially damaging information about their personal and professional

lives. This information had nothing to do with patients, but rather reflected on the nurses themselves. In the final report, the researchers disclosed their "confessions" in such a way that those reading the report could have identified the nurses who were involved.

5. A teacher of research and a student worked jointly on a research project. The teacher designed the project, analyzed most of the data, and wrote most of the conclusions. The student worked on the literature review, collected data, helped with the analysis, and discussed the interpretation with the teacher. When the article was published in a research journal, the teacher cited the student as second author.

6. This research project studied families who were experiencing the dying process a second time with a child whose sibling had died previously of the same disease (e.g., muscular dystrophy, Tay-Sachs disease). The nurse researcher spent many hours with the families and was included in intimate conferences with ministers, rabbis, physicians, family members, and close friends. Thus, the nurse was privy to much information of a personal and sensitive nature. As a result, the nurse constantly assessed who she shared information with, and she evaluated the nature and usefulness of this information.

7. A study on cancer patients' perceptions of radiation, chemotherapy, and surgery was funded by the American Cancer Society. This source of funding was not noted on the myriad of publications that resulted from the study.

8. In a study on care of mentally retarded children in a cluster home, the nurse carefully told the staff of the purpose and methods of the proposed research. When the research was completed the researcher found that there were some glaring deficiencies in the care of these children. For example, children with severe retardation were often left in uncomfortable positions for hours at a time and were rarely offered fluids; diapers were changed infrequently. Although the researcher was concerned as to how her findings would be received, she did report them accurately and completely.

9. A nurse researcher published a study on ostomy care in a journal read by nurses practicing in clinical areas. An ostomy nurse specialist took issue with the findings and wrote a caustic letter to the journal, which was subsequently published. The researcher, believing her findings had been misinterpreted, wrote a letter of response to the journal and requested it be published.

10. Three nurses on a critical care unit studied the use of relaxation therapy with (1) patients with a history of angina, (2) patients with myocardial infarction, and (3) patients with recent cardiac bypasses. Although their findings were "statistically significant" and suggested areas for nurse intervention that could improve patient care, they chose not to publish their findings, saying "We don't have the time" and "We know the results and that's what really matters."

Answers to be found at the back of the book.

Discussion Guidelines

In a small group, discuss what you would do to resolve the dilemma represented in each vignette.

The Rights to Full Disclosure

All research subjects, including patients, families, physicians, and nurses, are entitled to full disclosure about the research. They should be aware of the following aspects of any study:

1. The nature, duration, and purposes of a study
2. The methods, procedures, and processes by which data will be collected; presented in lay terminology
3. The use to which findings will be applied
4. Any and all inconveniences, potential harm, or discomforts that might be expected, including becoming a target for inclusion in future studies, risking loss of privacy or confidentiality, and commitment of personal unreimbursed time
5. Any results or side effects that might follow from participation in a study, including follow-up interviews or questionnaires

Directions

Read the following vignettes. Apply the questions provided in the Discussion Guidelines to each vignette.

1. A nurse researcher told the nurses on an intensive care unit that she was studying nurse–patient interaction by participant observation and interviews. The study would take 3 months and would be written up for publication. No harm or discomfort was expected, but if the nurses were "uncomfortable," they could choose not to be interviewed or "watched"; that is, no documentation regarding their interaction would go into the field notes. Data would be confidential, and all participants would be anonymous.

2. This 12-month study will examine the effect of patient education on cardiac rehabilitation patients. The purpose is to ascertain if education helps improve patient well-being and patient self-care techniques (e.g., less smoking, better diet, more exercise). The findings will be presented to the hospital staff and involved patients and will be written for publication. No discomfort or inconveniences are expected. Participation is voluntary. No negative results or side effects are expected.

3. While assessing patients for kidney dialysis and recognizing that there was a shortage of dialysis machines, so only certain patients could be dialyzed, a researcher decided to study patient compliance. Those patients who were compliant with the diet, taking medications, and so forth were felt to be more deserving of dialysis because they would probably live longer due to compliant behavior. The research protocol was presented as a study of patient compliance, but the underlying "use" of the research findings was not mentioned. The researcher believed that awareness of the real reason for the study would alter subjects' behavior. The study was presented as a study of compliance—patients filled in weekly questionnaires and documented when they did or

did not follow doctors' or nurses' orders. Patients were told the study would last for 2 months, that side effects were unexpected, and that the risks were negligible.

4. A nurse researcher was studying anorexia/bulimia in female college students. At the end of the study, which was clearly explained to them on a cover sheet of a packet of questionnaires, the subjects' names were given to a subject pool, meaning they could be contacted for future research. This possibility was not discussed with the subjects.

5. A nurse researcher wanted to get medical patients' perceptions of nursing care. In a clear explanation to the patients of the purposes, methods, and use of the research, the nurse indicated each interview would take about 10 minutes. However, each interview took more than 1 hour because the nurse subsequently thought of more questions to ask.

6. A nurse studying sexual needs of senior citizens realized, after data analysis, that she needed information for several additional questions. She decided to recontact the subject to gain the information she wanted.

Discussion Guidelines

After reading the vignettes, ask yourself the following questions.

1. Were any of the five principles of disclosure violated?
2. If so, which ones?
3. How were they violated?
4. How could you remedy the violation?

The Right of Self-Determination

The right of self-determination means that research subjects who give informed consent have full knowledge about the research in which they are participating and feel free from constraint or coercion of any kind when giving that consent. Coercive or seductive language in introduction letters and consent forms is therefore unacceptable and unethical.

Directions

Read the following letters. If necessary, rewrite the introduction letter and the consent form so that the subject's right of self-determination is not violated.

Introduction Letter

Dear Subject:

You are about to embark on a new and exciting experience, one which is expected to benefit you by reducing your pain and making the experience of birth more pleasurable and emotionally satisfying.

We are offering you wonder drug #1, to be administered intramuscularly when you feel contractions are painful enough to warrant pain medication.

We look forward to having you participate with us, your health care team, in this new endeavor, which we expect will be a major contribution to the practice of obstetrics.

Sincerely,

Informed Consent

I, _____, a patient on the cardiac care unit, agree to participate in a bathing study. I know I will have 3 days of conventional bed baths and 3 days of Totman towel baths and will be asked to evaluate the baths. I recognize that there are no known risks for me and that there are no personal benefits because the study is to evaluate the effects of the different baths on cardiac activity and patient comfort. However, if a particular type of bath is found (1) to be more comfortable or (2) to interfere less with normal cardiac activity, such recognition could have implications for improving nursing care of patients in the cardiac intensive care unit.

Discussion Guidelines

Answer the following questions with a group of fellow students or colleagues.

1. What changes did you make to either or both letters?
2. Why?
3. Are there any areas in either letter that require further explanation?

The Rights of Privacy, Anonymity, and Confidentiality

All research subjects have the rights of **privacy**, **anonymity**, and **confidentiality**. The definitions of these are often misinterpreted. A clear understanding of each concept is necessary so that nurse researchers or practicing nurses aware of ongoing research can evaluate if the rights of privacy, anonymity, and confidentiality are being violated.

Definitions

Directions

Match the letter of the correct definition to the appropriate word at the left. Place your answers in the space provided.

_____ 1. Confidentiality

_____ 2. Privacy

_____ 3. Anonymity

A. This enables a person to behave and think without interference or concern that her or his behavior or thoughts may be used to embarrass or demean the person later.

B. This concept applies when even the investigator cannot link a subject with the information reported. The best method to maintain this concept is the use of code numbers in lieu of real names, keeping the actual list under lock and key in a separate place.

C. This means that any information that a subject divulges will not be made public or available to anyone.

Examples of Violations

Directions

Put the letter of each of the following examples to the left of the concept that it violates.

_____ 1. Confidentiality

_____ 2. Privacy

_____ 3. Anonymity

A. In a study of patients with arthritis the researcher used real names in her field notes.

B. In a study of nurses rating weekend versus weekday work schedules, the researcher permitted nursing administrators to examine the raw data.

C. The patient was afraid that what he said in the questionnaire would be used against him, affecting his care.

Answers to be found at back of the book.

Discussion Guidelines

In a group discuss the correct answers to the definitions and examples of violations. Discuss how each concept—confidentiality, privacy, anonymity—could be violated in some other research projects that you are aware of or that you make up.

Keeping Research Subjects Free From Harm

All research studies that involve human subjects should be closely examined to ensure that subjects are not at risk. As patient advocates, nurses must always have the protection of patients uppermost in their minds.

Directions

Read the research studies in the references.

Discussion Guidelines

Discuss the following questions with your fellow students or colleagues.

1. What are the potential risks of each project?
2. What could be done to minimize the risks?

References

Draucker, C. (1991). The healing process of female adult incest survivors: Constructing a personal residence. *Image: Journal of Nursing Scholarship*, 24(1), 4–8.

Gift, A., Moore, T., & Soeken, K. (1992). Relaxation to reduce dyspnea and anxiety in COPD patients. *Nursing Research*, 41(4), 242–246.

Harrison, L., Leeper, J., & Yoon, M. (1991). Preterm infants' physiologic responses to early parent touch. *Western Journal of Nursing Research*, 13(6), 698–713.

Hartweg, D. (1993). Self-care actions of healthy middle-age women to promote well-being. *Nursing Research*, 42(4), 221–227.

Keithley, J., Zeller, J., Szeluga, D., & Urbanski, P. (1992). National alterations in persons with HIV infection. *Image: Journal of Nursing Scholarship*, 24(3), 183–187.

Sherrod, R. (1991). Obstetrical role strain for male nursing students. *Western Journal of Nursing Research*, 13(4), 494–502.

Human Subjects' Consent Form

 Different types of research have different requirements for the participation of human subjects. These requirements must be spelled out clearly in a **consent form**. The following nine elements of consent should be present in human subject consent forms:

1. **Purpose/Introduction** What is being studied? Why? Why me?
2. **Procedures** What will happen to me if I participate that would not otherwise happen to me?
3. **Risks/Discomforts**
4. **Benefits**
5. **Alternatives** Therapeutic or treatment options in lieu of participation
6. **Questions** Plan the time for a later discussion
7. **Experimental Subjects' Bill of Rights** Present to subject
8. **Payment** Is there any?
9. **Signatures** Subject, including parents if child is involved, and investigators

Directions

Read the following five abstracts, and write a consent form, "Consent to Be a Research Subject," that includes the nine elements for each research project.

Abstract

Title: Preterm Infants' Physiologic Response to Early Parent Touch

Nurses working in neonatal intensive care units (NICUs) are concerned with promoting parent-infant attachment and generally acknowledge the importance of encouraging parents to hold and touch their infants. However, as a result of recent studies indicating that excessive handling may cause hypoxia in preterm infants, many nurses are reluctant to encourage parents to touch their infants in the NICU. Yet no previous studies have examined the specific effects of early parent touch on young preterm infants. The purpose of this study was to determine whether preterm infants' physiologic responses to parental touch during NICU visits are influenced by their gestational age, birth weight, gender, behavioral state, or morbidity status, by the use of supplemental oxygen, by the amounts of tactile stimulation during the 2 hours preceding parent visits, or by the amount of parent and nurse touch during visits. This study was part of a larger research project designed to (a) describe the physical characteristics of touch used by parents in touching their preterm infants and (b) determine the effects of parent touch on the heart rates and arterial oxygen saturation levels of preterm infants. Other results from the larger study are reported elsewhere (Harrison, Leeper, & Yoon, 1990).

Source: Harrison, L. L., Leeper, J., & Yoon, M. (1991). Preterm infants' physiologic responses to early parent touch. *Western Journal of Nursing Research, 13*(6), 698–713.

Abstract

Title: Nutritional Alterations in Persons with HIV Infection

Potential relationships among nutritional status, immune function, and quality of life were examined in a convenience sample of 40 outpatient homosexual and bisexual males stratified into five categories, using modified Walter Reed Staging Criteria. Nutritional status was assessed by measuring height, weight, triceps skinfold thickness, arm circumference, nutrient intake, and serum albumin. Immune status was evaluated by determining T-helper cell numbers and percentages. The Quality of Life test was used to obtain information about life quality. Nutritional assessment failed to show significant differences among groups with the exception that serum albumin levels were reduced in persons with AIDS. The significance of change in serum albumin in regard to nutritional status is unclear since serum albumin is affected by a number of nonnutritional factors, such as hydration status and liver function. The study also revealed a significant decline in T-helper percentages, but not absolute T-helper cell numbers as a function of disease stage. There were no statistically significant differences between the quality of life scores with respect to each grouping. These data suggest that symptomatic patients as well as those with ARC or stable AIDS are able to maintain body weight and composition.

Source: Keithley, J. K., Zeller, J. M., Szeluga, D. J., & Urbanski, P. A. (1992). Nutritional alterations in persons with HIV infection. *Image: Journal of Nursing Scholarship* 24(3), 183–187.

Abstract

Title: Temperature and Temperature Measurement After Induced Hypothermia

This study was designed to assess factors associated with afterdrop, the fall in core temperature following completion of cardiac surgery, and determine the validity of noninvasive measures of temperature to predict core temperature in the severely hypothermic patient. Twenty-five postcardiac surgery patients served as subjects. Core temperature was measured using the pulmonary artery, bladder, and esophageal sites. The less invasive measures included a tympanic membrane thermometer, oral and axillary electronic thermometers, and a forehead surface temperature indicator. Temperatures were recorded every 10 minutes for 2 hours. End-of-surgery temperatures ranged from 30.3-38.3°C (86.5-100.9°F) with a mean of 36.02°C (96.84°F). Temperature change over the next hour ranged from a rise of 2.5°C (4.5°F) to a fall of 4.1°C (7.2°F). Factors associated with afterdrop included age, end-of-surgery temperature (both positively), and body mass (negatively). No noninvasive measure appeared to be a valid indicator of core temperature in these hypothermic patients.

Source: Heidenreich, T., Giuffre, M., & Doorley, J. (1992). Temperature and temperature measurement after induced hypothermia. *Nursing Research*, 41(5), 296–300.

Abstract

Title: Human Sexuality in Adults with Insulin-Dependent Diabetes Mellitus

This qualitative study was conducted to explore human sexuality in adults with insulin-dependent diabetes mellitus. Data from interviews of 11 men and women were used to formulate a substantive theory describing the process of changes in sexuality that occur in adults with this chronic illness. The core category of the theory is transforming, which is supported by the subcategories of valuing self and meeting intimacy needs. Information from the study can be used in nursing to provide client care, teaching, and counseling for adults with insulin-dependent diabetes mellitus.

Source: LeMone, P. (1993). Human sexuality in adults with insulin-diabetes mellitus. *Image: Journal of Nursing Scholarship, 25*(2), 101–105.

Abstract

Title: The Effect of Thermal Biofeedback and Progressive Muscle Relaxation Training in Reducing Blood Pressure of Patients with Essential Hypertension

In order to assess the effectiveness of the thermal biofeedback training combined with the progressive muscle relaxation therapy in the treatment of patients with essential hypertension, blood pressure decline was measured on the treatment group who had the combined thermal biofeedback and progressive muscle relaxation training (n=11), and on the control group who had only the progressive muscle relaxation training (n=8). Baseline blood pressure was measured four times for two weeks on both groups. For the treatment group, blood pressure was measured twice before and after each of eight sessions of thermal biofeedback training for four weeks. For the control group, blood pressure was measured every two visits to a clinic for progressive muscle relaxation self-training twice before and after the self-training. A significant decline of the systolic blood pressure by 20.6 mmHg and of the diastolic blood pressure by 14.4 mmHg was observed in the treatment group. There was a tendency for both blood pressures to increase in the control group.

Source: Hahn, Y. B., Ro, Y. J., Song, H. H., Kim, N. C., Kim, H. S., & Yoo, Y. S. (1993). The effect of thermal biofeedback and progressive muscle relaxation training in reducing blood pressure of patients with essential hypertension. *Image: Journal of Nursing Scholarship, 25*(3), 204–207.

Assessing a Research Subject's Statement of Consent

Individual **consent forms** are vitally important in most nursing research and should contain the nine elements listed in the previous exercise.

Directions

Read the following hypothetical statement of consent, and follow the discussion guidelines.

Discussion Guidelines

1. Which of the essential nine elements of consent are present or absent in this consent form?
2. Rewrite the consent form to include all nine elements.

Human Subject Consent Form

Date:_____

I, _____, consent to participate in a nursing study being conducted by Ms. M. Susan, RN, MSN, CS, that compares two methods of measuring my activity tolerance. I understand that several tests will be made to determine my activity tolerance, but the results will have no effect on my present nursing care. This has been verified by my physician, Dr. AHN and is being conducted with her approval.

Both methods have been explained to me by Ms. Susan, and I understand what will happen to me if I participate. I have been assured that my anonymity, privacy and confidentiality will be honored and maintained. I have also been assured that there are no risks or side effects to me by virtue of being involved in this study. I agree to participate in this study and understand that I may withdraw from it at any time.

Signature:_____

Witness: _____   Date:_____

20 Minimizing Risks to Human Subjects—Calculating the Risk: Benefit Ratio in Nursing Research

  Risks to research subjects in clinical studies should be weighed against the potential benefits to them and/or to society in the knowledge produced. The benefits should exceed the risks.

Directions

Read the following vignettes. The questions provided in the Discussion Guidelines should be applied to each vignette.

1. A neonatologist wants to use different new antibiotics to fight infection in critically ill newborns. He has a control group, which receives a traditional antibiotic, and two experimental groups, which receive different types of new antibiotics. Babies are randomly selected for the three groups. Parental consent is not sought when a baby is placed in the experimental group.

2. A researcher wants to conduct some blood studies on patients receiving chemotherapy. The research protocol requires that the patients have blood drawn at certain intervals over the 2-week time limit. The question of who would pay for this additional lab work was not discussed in the proposal that went to the **Institutional Review Board** (IRB).

3. A nurse researcher was planning to conduct a study on nurse–nurse interaction in a critical care unit. This study was approved by the IRB. During the data-collection process, the nurse was able to collect considerable data on nurse–physician relationships and decided to present and publish this information as well.

4. A psychiatrist wanted to study the effects of prolixin administered intramuscularly on psychoses. He planned to give one group of psychiatric patients prolixin intramuscularly every 72 hours (common practice) and give another group prolixin every 36 hours over a one-week period. Psychotic patients would be randomly assigned to one group or the other. The psychiatrist did not plan to get consent from the patients ("They are too sick to decide") or families ("Many of these patients' families could not make an educated decision").

5. A nurse researcher is studying nursing practice in a high-risk labor and delivery room with the hope that her observations will lead to suggested interventions for improving patient care or at least to greater understanding of labor and delivery nursing. As a participant observer, she is privy to women patients who are in various stages of distress, who are naked, and who occasionally lose their composure.

6. Mr. J is dying of Lou Gehrig's disease. A nurse researcher believes a certain diet will be helpful in curing the disease. The diet is high in fat, low in protein and carbohydrates. The nurse researcher and a nutritionist present a research proposal to the IRB that would put Mr. J on this diet for a certain period of time. Then the progress of the disease would be evaluated and a decision made whether to continue the diet.

7. A nurse researcher is a participant observer in a self-help group of impaired nurses, all of whom have problems with drugs or alcohol. The researcher wants their full names, addresses, and places of employment, and educational histories for research purposes.
8. A nurse researcher is studying touch with the elderly. She plans to touch a certain group of patients in a nursing home every hour for about 1 minute. A control group of patients will not be touched.

Discussion Guidelines

Respond to the following questions for each vignette.

1. How important is the research?
2. What are the benefits?
3. What are the risks?
4. As a member of the IRB, would you vote that this research be given approval or not? If not, what (if anything) could the researcher do to make the study acceptable and ethical?
5. Choose one of the following categories of risk that characterizes each vignette.
   a. No positive or negative effects expected on the research subjects
   b. Temporary discomfort, anxiety, or physical pain
   c. Unusual levels of temporary discomfort that may last beyond the end of the study and that require a debriefing interview or conference to relieve a subject of undue anxiety
   d. Risks of permanent damage
   e. Certainty of permanent damage

21

Finding the Philosophy of Science in Famous Quotations

The following quotations from well-known writers on the philosophy of science reveal either the **positivistic** (P) or **naturalistic/interpretive** (NI) perspective.

Directions

Place a P or NI on the line to the left of each of the following statements.

_____ 1. "We should set aside all previous habits of thought, see through and break down the mental barriers which these habits have set along the horizons of our thinking and in full . . . freedom, proceed and lay hold of those genuine problems still awaiting fresh formulation which the liberated horizons on all sides disclose to us . . . " (Husserl, 1960; p. 34).

_____ 2. "Underneath the visible edifices of the human world there is a hidden, invisible structure of interests and forces waiting to be uncovered by the researcher. The manifest is not the whole story; latency is there to be studied. Or, in the simplest terms, the world is not what it appears to be" (Berger and Kellner, 1981; p. 4).

_____ 3. "Human phenomena don't speak for themselves; they must be interpreted . . . A deviation of the act of interpretation was at the center of Max Weber's methodology" (Berger and Kellner, 1981; p. 10).

_____ 4. "All human situations carry meaning—if one prefers, are illuminated by meaning from within themselves. The purpose of sociological interpretation is to bring out these meanings and meaning system" (Berger and Kellner, 1981; p. 40).

_____ 5. "In this philosophy, the scientific attitude is applied not only to the sciences, but also to human affairs. Science is confined to the observable and manipulatable" (Lacey, 1976).

_____ 6. "The scientific method is considered the one and only process for scientific discovery, experimental quantitative research methodology and design" (Watson, 1981).

_____ 7. "Science is the pursuit of truth" (Schlick, 1932).

Answers to be found at the back of the book.

Discussion Guidelines

Discuss the following questions in a group of fellow students or colleagues.

1. Do you disagree with any of the answers? Why?
2. Do you agree with the answers? Why?

References

Berger, P., & Kellner, H. (1981). *Sociology Reinterpreted*. New York: Anchor Books.

Husserl, E. (1960). *Ideas*. New York: Collier Books.

Lacey, A. R. (1976). *A Dictionary of Philosophy*. New York: Charles Scribner's Sons.

Schlick, M. (1932). The future of philosophy. In P. A. Schipp (Ed.), *College of the Pacific Publications in Philosophy*. Stockton, CA: University of the Pacific.

Watson, J. (1981). Nursing's scientific quest. *Nurse Outlook*, July, 29(7), 413–416.

Philosophy of Science in Nursing Research

Two schools of thought are the basis for most nursing research questions and procedures—the **positivist** tradition (P) and the **naturalistic/interpretive** (N/I) tradition. The following statements reflect the beliefs of one or the other of these research philosophies.

Directions

Reread the Introduction for this Part and the definitions of positivist and naturalistic/interpretive in the glossary. Place a P or NI on the line to the left of each of the following statements.

_____ 1. Fundamental differences exist between the natural, or physical, sciences and the psychosocial sciences that require different methodologies for each.

_____ 2. Scientists can and do attain objective knowledge of both the psychosocial and the physical worlds.

_____ 3. Research that studies the whole person must take into account both the historic dimension of human action and the subjective aspects of human experience.

_____ 4. There is no one objective reality waiting to be measured.

_____ 5. The logic of inquiry and research procedures should be the same whether you are studying people or plants.

_____ 6. Social order in the universe is relatively mechanistic.

_____ 7. If scientists are to really comprehend people, they must come to understand each person's own definition of his or her reality.

_____ 8. Objectivity in research can be obtained by setting forth your formal research design.

_____ 9. Social order is constantly in a state of becoming. Therefore, scientists cannot impose fixed, rigid categories on a social world that is constantly in the process of evolution.

Answers to be found at the back of the book.

Discussion Guidelines

After you have completed the exercise, discuss the following questions in small groups. Obtain feedback from a teacher or knowledgeable colleague regarding your understanding.

1. Which of the two research traditions more closely reflects your beliefs? Why?
2. Think about what you believe to be "true." Are your beliefs close to the positivist or naturalistic/interpretive philosophy?

23 Categorize the Philosophic Perspective in Nursing Studies

The following excerpts from published nursing research articles in nursing literature can be categorized as either **positivistic** (P) or **naturalistic/interpretive** (NI) perspectives.

Directions

Place a P or NI on the line to the left of each of the following study descriptions.

_____ 1. A study conducted by Hutchinson (1992), entitled "Nurses Who Violate the Nurse Practice Act: Transformation of Professional Identity," states: "The purpose of this research was to explore and describe the experiences of nurses who had been accused of violating the Nurse Practice Act." The goal of this study was to understand the experience of nurses involved in investigations and hearings in response to their violations. The methods of research were interviews, participant observation, and document analysis.

_____ 2. In a study entitled "After the Casualties: Vietnam Nurses' Identities and Career Decisions" (Norman, 1992), the author elicits wartime experiences of 50 nurses through taped interviews. Results indicate that the nurses' responsibilities in stateside hospitals often seemed diminished and patient needs distinct from those of battle casualties. Findings confirm that the nurses' postwar reactions were similar to those of other wars. Career choices of most of the nurses were altered by their wartime experience.

_____ 3. The abstract of the study by Lowe (1993), "Maternal Confidence for Labor: Development of the Childbirth Self-Efficacy Inventory," states "The Childbirth Self-Efficacy Inventory (CBSEI) is a self-report instrument that measures outcome expectancies and self-efficacy expectancies for coping with an approaching childbirth experience."

_____ 4. In the study "Decision Making by Patients with Breast Cancer: The Role of Information in Treatment Selection," Hughes (1993) found that "subjects' choice of treatment was unrelated to the amount of information they received during the clinic visit. Manner of presentation also did not influence treatment selection. However, treatment selection was related to the amount of information subjects received prior to their clinic visit ($p < 0.01$)."

_____ 5. Redfern and Hutchinson (1994), in their study entitled "Women's Experiences of Repeatedly Contracting Sexually Transmitted Diseases", explored and described women's experiences of repetitively contracting sexually transmitted diseases (STDs). The method of research used was interviews with 8 women along with "stories and anecdotes from one author's clinical practice."

_____ 6. The study "Newborn Behavioral Performance in Colic and Non-colic Infants" by Covington et al. (1991), incorporates the Brazelton Neonatal Behavior Assessment Scale (BNBAS) in its investigation. This investigation produced evidence of significant and measurable difference in the behavioral performance of the two infant groups.

Answers to be found at the back of the book.

Discussion Guidelines

Discuss the following questions in a group of colleagues or fellow students.

1. Do you agree with the answers given in the key? If so, why? If not, why not?
2. Look again at the vignettes. Note that some report research methods, some report research purpose, and some report research findings. Discuss how the philosophic perspective is revealed in these different parts of a research study.

References

Covington, C., Croenwett, L., & Loveland-Cherry, C. (1991). Newborn behavioral performance in colic and non-colic infants. *Nursing Research*, *40*(5), 292–297.

Hughes, K. K. (1993). Decision making by patients with breast cancer: The role of information in treatment selection. *Oncology Nursing Forum*, *20*(5), 623–628.

Hutchinson, S. A. (1992). Nurses who violate the nurse practice act: Transformation of professional identity. *Image: Journal of Nursing Scholarship*, *4*(2), 133–139.

Lowe, N. K. (1993). Maternal confidence for labor: Development of the childbirth self-efficacy inventory. *Research in Nursing and Health*, *16*(2), 141–149.

Norman, E. M. (1992). After the casualities: Vietnam nurses' identities and career decisions. *Nursing Research*, *41*(2), 110–113.

Redfern, N., & Hutchinson, S. (1994). Women's Experiences of Repeatedly Contracting Sexually Transmitted Diseases, *Health Care for Women International*. Vol. 15, 423–433

24

Theoretical and Philosophic Bases of Inquiry

  Research critiquing should not be viewed as merely a cookbook exercise. Instead, nurse critics, in order to fully understand and carry out their role, should be aware of certain scientific principles that influence their thinking when they prepare a research critique. This exercise will familiarize you with the principles suggested for "good" science and with the dichotomous beliefs held by nurses who come from different scientific traditions.

Directions

Match the principles of science on the right with the nursing research beliefs on the left. Each principle can be matched to two different beliefs, or schools of thought. Put the corresponding letter in the space provided at the left.

Beliefs

_____ 1. These researchers concede that there is a degree of order in the world, but stress its changing and complex nature. They believe that humans interpret and shape their own reality.

_____ 2. These nurse scientists define **theory** in rigorous terms that are applicable only to systems involving sets of **postulates** from which testable **hypotheses** can be derived. These researchers emphasize theory over **data** (observations).

_____ 3. Some researchers use artificial or scientific language systems to avoid the perceived inadequacies of ordinary language. **Deductive** hypothesis-testing studies use this language as they define key terms as they go through the process of testing the hypotheses.

_____ 4. These nurse researchers argue that a fixed, stable order characterizes social as well as physical reality. They expect to uncover

Principles

A. The nature and adequacy of proof

B. The nature of reality

C. The value of natural or artificial language

D. The relationship between theory and data

E. The observer's relationship to observed phenomena

F. Selection of units of analysis and sources of data

"what actually exists." They believe that humans respond, adapt, or cope with physical and social forces.

_____ 5. These researchers believe observers should be able to distance themselves and make unbiased observations. They value strategies or instruments designed to eliminate observer bias.

_____ 6. These nurse investigators aim for **probability sampling** procedures and randomization of selection, if possible.

_____ 7. These researchers contend that the observer always influences and is influenced by the reality under investigation. They emphasize being aware and reporting on the subjective, interpretive nature of the observer–observed interaction.

_____ 8. These nurse scientists believe that only logically related statements explaining an investigator's observations or making them meaningful can be considered a scientific theory in a broad sense. These researchers stress observation (data).

_____ 9. These researchers, using more natural language, believe science should be **inductive**, extracting out of nature (data) a conceptual explanation.

_____10. a. These nurse scientists advocate the rigid adoption of measurement and statistical rules used in the physical sciences.

b. These nurses believe a theory must be predictive.

c. These nurses believe **validity** and **reliability** measures are necessary to validate measurement techniques.

11. a. These nurse investigators believe that the application of measurement and statistical-rules and procedures to complex, interactional human systems is not appropriate, but needs more methodological research

b. These nurses believe a theory should promote understanding.

c. These nurses believe that standard techniques for establishing validity and reliability are inappropriate and reductionistic, sacrificing generality for specificity.

_____12. These nurse investigators are concerned with **theoretical sampling** rather than **random sampling**. That is, their sampling process may change during the research process depending on empirical behaviors they observe and the **concepts** they discover. They aim for depth of data.

Answers to be found at the back of the book.

Discussion Guidelines

Discuss your answers with a group of fellow students or colleagues, and consider the following questions:

1. Where do you stand on each principle?
2. Which scientific tradition is most appealing to you? Why?
3. How will your approach influence your critiques of research studies and proposals?

PART 3

Understanding and Evaluating Nursing Research

✢ Understanding the Language of Science

If nurses are to apply research findings in practice, we must all be prepared to read, understand, and intelligently evaluate the published and presented reports of studies. It should not be necessary to become a career scientist yourself to understand the format of a scientific article, to become literate in research terminology, and to interpret tables and graphs. This book's application exercises offer guided opportunities to master these skills, as well as skills in identifying researchable problems, judging study designs, and conducting a formal critique.

Typical Format of a Research Article

Almost all reports of nursing studies published in journals are written in a somewhat standardized format. The typical sections would be arranged as follows:

1. **Abstract**   This section summarizes the key points as briefly as possible, including purpose, objectives or hypotheses, study participants or sample members, data-collection and analysis procedures, and the important findings.
2. **Introduction**   This section relates the study to prior knowledge by reviewing previous theoretical and research literature and by stating the specific goals or purposes of the current study.
3. **Method**   This section explains in detail how the study was conducted so that it could be replicated by someone else. This section should describe the subjects or sample members and how they were obtained, the type of design or organizational plan for conducting the study, and the data collection instruments and procedures for analyzing the data once they are collected.
4. **Results**   This section relates the outcome of the study. Results often are presented in tables and graphs and include the outcome of statistical tests used on the data.
5. **Discussion**   This section explains what the results mean with regard to the study purpose and relates them to the theoretical framework.
6. **References**   These should include books and articles that provide important background for the study.

Basic Research Terminology

Knowledge of the specialized terminology likely to be encountered in a scientific article is mandatory. The following are some key terms basic to understanding any study report. Look up the meaning for each in the Glossary at the back of the book.

Concept	Instruments
Operational definition	Reliability
Variable	Validity
Independent variable	Population
Dependent variable	Sample
Extraneous variable	The Hawthorne effect
Confounding variable	The halo effect
Hypothesis	Double-blind method
Data	Field research
	Grounded theory
	Qualitative study

Common research symbols should also be recognized. Examples appear on the end papers of this book.

Steps in the Research Process

If developing theories and verifying them are the goals of science, the research process is the tool of science. By definition, research is a process that takes place in a series of steps representing the general line of thinking that investigators consider when conducting a study. For the purpose of clarity and comprehensiveness, our list of steps consists of ten modular, mobile, and flexible stages as follows:

1. Stating a research question or problem
2. Defining the purpose of the study
3. Reviewing related literature
4. Formulating **hypotheses** and defining **variables**
5. Selecting the research design
6. Selecting the **population**, **sample**, and **setting**
7. Conducting a **pilot study**
8. Collecting the **data**
9. Analyzing the data
10. Communicating conclusions

Refer to the glossary at the end of this guidebook to familiarize yourself with the fundamental tasks associated with each of the preceding steps.

✜ Study Designs: Blueprints for Research

Study designs are basically a set of instructions or a plan that tells an investigator or a reader how and from whom data are to be collected, and how it will be analyzed in order to answer a specified research question. Sometimes study designs are called the **protocol** for the research and include a timetable that spells out what and when procedures or operations will be done.

Types of Studies According to Purpose of Design

Most nursing research has one of five major purposes and is designed specifically to accomplish it. These purposes also serve as a way to classify or categorize types of nursing studies. The five types of nursing studies, their purposes and methods are summarized below in the Table.

Type of Design	Purpose	Methods
Exploratory	To obtain insights as a basis for future research	Interviews, case studies, observations
Descriptive	To obtain complete and accurate information about a phenomenon	Questionnaires, surveys, analysis of records
Explanatory	To provide conceptual analysis grounded in observation of human behavior	Constant comparative analysis, participant observation
Experimental and quasi-experimental	To test hypotheses about relationships	Experiments, quasi-experiments
Methodological	To develop or refine a new research technique or procedure	Validity and reliability tests

Purposes of Study Designs

Researchers select their plan or design to serve two major purposes: (1) To answer the research question as validly, objectively, accurately, and economically as possible and (2) To control the **extraneous** or **error variances** (other factors that might confound the results).

The Research Consumer's Role

As a consumer of research findings, your role is to recognize what kind of study design was used, whether it was well-suited to the problem under investigation, and what its advantages and disadvantages were, given the way it was implemented. This requires familiarity with a few essential points about each type of study design.

Study Design Essentials

HISTORICAL STUDY DESIGNS   The purpose of **historical study designs** is to explain the past and its implications for the present and future by systematically collecting, evaluating, and interpreting evidence from the past (maps, books, artifacts, diaries, public documents, photographs, and the like). The major advantage of historical research is in its potential to illuminate a current question through intensive study of selected materials that already exist.

The major disadvantages include the following:

1. The investigator must rely on sources that already exist without being able to ask clarifying questions or fill in gaps.
2. The investigator must be able to translate the language and ideas in terms of their historical context and period.
3. The investigator is unable to accurately predict a timetable for completion of a study because it is difficult to calculate what might be involved in locating **primary sources** (first-hand information) and **secondary sources** (second-hand or third-hand accounts) relevant to the study question.

The value of historical study can be determined by asking the two key questions:

1. Are the data sources genuine or authentic?
2. Is the information contained in them and the researcher's interpretation of its meaning accurate or correct?

CASE STUDY DESIGNS   **Case study designs** provide in-depth analyses of a single subject (an individual patient, a family, a hospital ward, or a professional organization) in order to gain insight, provide background information for more controlled and broader studies, develop explanations of human processes, and provide rich, descriptive anecdotes.

The advantages of case study designs are as follows:

1. They offer a researcher insight into little known problems that can provide a basis for the planning of future studies.
2. They can suggest hypotheses or directions for future research.
3. They are well-suited to learning about a process over time. For example, Freud's psychoanalytic theory was developed over a long series of case studies of psychiatric patients in Vienna.

The disadvantages of case study designs are as follows:

1. Researchers have no guidelines to help them decide how much data is enough.
2. The cost-effectiveness and objectivity of data obtained over a relatively long period of time from one subject or data source is open to question.
3. Researchers can neither test causal hypotheses (cause-and-effect relationships) nor be certain about how far results based on case studies can be generalized to others.

Evaluating the worth of case study designs requires that you decide if the ambiguity necessary to gather a rich array of data to arrive at insights justifies the lack of rigor and conventional control.

SURVEY RESEARCH DESIGNS   **Survey research designs**, also called **nonexperimental designs,** can use large or small groups, questionnaires or interviews, and can serve descriptive, comparative, correlational, developmental, and evaluative purposes. Their distinguishing characteristic is that they involve collecting information from a variety of sample subjects and generalizing the findings to the **population** of interest. Survey studies are well-suited to collecting demographic information, social characteristics, behavioral patterns, and information bases and are very popular in nursing research studies.

The advantage of a survey design is that it combines flexibility of content and purpose with elements of precision and control. It can be used to gather information from a large number of subjects with minimal expenditure of time and money. It is relatively easy to replicate or repeat, keeping features and procedures unchanged. It can take advantage of existing standardized scales and questionnaires.

Disadvantages of survey designs include the following:

1. Low return rates from mailed surveys because of their impersonality.
2. The possibility that prestructured questions are irrelevant or confusing.
3. The tendency of data to be relatively superficial because cause-and-effect relationships about study variables are not included.

Evaluating the merit of survey designs involves establishing their **validity** (Does the study measure what it is supposed to?), **reliability** (Do instruments for data collection provide consistent results?), objectivity (Are sources of error eliminated as much as possible?), relevance and significance, overall credibility (believability according to the canons of scientific methods), and efficiency in view of results obtained.

EXPERIMENTAL STUDY DESIGNS   The term *experiment* sometimes is used synonymously or interchangeably with the term *research project* or *study*. In the language of science, **experiment** has a very precise and specific meaning. It refers to a kind of study in which the researcher manipulates (controls) one or more **independent variables**, assigns subjects to either **experimental** or **control groups** on a chance (random) basis, initially selects the subjects (sample) on a random basis, and finally, observes the **dependent variable**, outcome, or effect that presumably is due to the independent variable.

The advantages of an experimental design are that an investigator can control **extraneous variance**, minimize error variance, and systematically make the experimental variance effects more obvious. The rigor and control of experimental study designs are also the only way researchers can establish cause-and-effect relationships, testing what in science are called *causal hypotheses*.

The disadvantages of experimental designs are that they are not always suitable for use under real-world, nursing conditions:

1. It is not always feasible or ethical to manipulate some variables if care or the standard of care would be denied to certain patients.
2. Random selection and equal treatment of experimental and control groups rarely occur under real-world conditions, even though they may be possible in a laboratory.
3. Many of the phenomena that are of concern to nursing are complex and multidimensional. Some authorities therefore believe that experimental designs, which are well-suited to studying relationships between two variables in the physical sciences, may be reductionistic and incompatible with the holistic philosophy of nursing.

Ex Post Facto Designs **Ex post facto designs** study something after the fact. For example, did 20 years of cigarette smoking cause cancer? Did taking drugs during pregnancy cause or become significantly correlated with birth defects? Did regular exercise or taking calcium postmenopause relate to a better health status in old age? Study samples for ex post facto designs are, in effect, self-selected because they share a common characteristic or experience.

The advantage of ex post facto studies is that they allow us to learn from the experience of others that which would be unethical to introduce as part of an experiment. The disadvantages are mainly due to weaknesses of an ex post facto design:

1. The researcher cannot establish cause and effect, only correlations.
2. The researcher cannot randomly assign subjects to experimental treatments.
3. The possibility for misinterpretations of study results is high.

It takes a sharp reader to recognize when a researcher has gone beyond ex post facto data in reporting a study's significance.

Methodological Study Designs **Methodological studies** are planned to develop tools, instruments, or methods that are appropriate for answering nursing research questions. Conducting these studies places nurse researchers at an advantage because research tools developed in other disciplines may not always suit nursing's purposes. The disadvantages, however, are associated with the tedious, time-consuming process of generating, validating, standardizing, and establishing the reliability of a measurement or investigational tool or device. Canons of validity and reliability are the primary criteria on which the outcome of a methodological study should be judged (See Glossary).

Strategies for Interpreting Visual Presentations of Data

Since results of studies are often presented in tables and graphs, you will need to know how to interpret them. The following list provides some methods for easier understanding of tables and graphs:

1. Try to spot trends (e.g., what is the most frequent score?).
2. Did the researcher pick the most appropriate measure of central tendency? (Note that the **mean** is the average; the **median** is the midpoint between the upper and lower halves of the scores in a data set; and the **mode** is the most common or typical score.)
3. Pay attention to the variability or range of scores in a data set. Sometimes scores are grouped together, and sometimes scores can be extremely different from each other. High variability indicates that a consensus or similarities may not have been found.
4. Look for exceptions and missing data.
5. Compare what is printed in tables with what is discussed in the text of the article. Watch for contradictions or inconsistencies.
6. Get in the habit of reading the captions or legends for tables and figures. They can help you understand what you are seeing.

✤ Conducting Formal Critiques of Scientific Reports and Proposals

As a practicing nurse and consumer of nursing research, you may be invited or even inclined to write a formal critique of a study proposal or report that you read or hear presented at a professional meeting. Scientific criticism means carefully reviewing, dissecting, analyzing, and evaluating the merit of a study based on the canons of science.

A good critique is not an exercise in nitpicking or censure, and it should be distinguishable from a study review, which only summarizes the major characteristics or features of a study without making a judgment about the study's scientific worth or merit. The critic's challenge is to determine what a researcher has tried to do and to evaluate the strategies used and the findings obtained, given the overall constraints of the conditions for the study. A good critique presents both the criteria for and the evidence of the judgments made. The ultimate purpose of a research critique is to help a researcher refine and improve a study based on an appraisal of its strengths and limitations, from the point of view of a practitioner who must rely on the findings to guide practice decisions. Exercises in this part will help you develop and sharpen the skills needed for conducting systematic critiques.

25 The Research Consumer's Role: Reviewing or Critiquing Nursing Research

Leaders in nursing agree that all nurses, regardless of their educational level, should be prepared with the essential skills for functioning in the role of research consumer. Research consumers should be able to review and *critique* nursing research. This exercise will help you learn the differences between a research review and a research critique.

Directions

Choose the correct answers from Column B and put the corresponding letter in the spaces provided for each statement in Column A.

Column A

_____ 1. "A critical estimate of a piece of research which has been carefully and systematically studied by a critic who has used specific criteria to appraise . . . the general features . . . " (Leininger, 1968)

_____ 2. Like a book report that summarizes the plot

_____ 3. Makes a judgement about the proposal or reports scientific merits and ultimate worth

_____ 4. Presents both criteria for and evidence of the judgements that are made

_____ 5. "Identifies and summarizes the major features and characteristics of a study" (Leininger, 1968)

_____ 6. Helps an investigator improve his or her program of inquiry

_____ 7. Helps research consumers decide how to use findings from a study

Column B

A. Research review
B. Research critique

Answers to be found at the back of the book.

Discussion Guidelines

Now that you are clear about the differences between a research review and a research critique, discuss the following questions with your colleagues or fellow students.

1. How are the process and end results of critiquing a research proposal or study similar to or different from using your critical skills in evaluating clinical practice problems?
2. If you had written a research proposal or study, would you prefer to be reviewed or critiqued by your colleagues? Why?
3. How can a research critique be useful to consumers? To practicing nurses?

Reference

Leininger, M. (1968). The research critique: Nature, function and art. In: *Communicating Nursing Research: The Research Critique*, pp. 20–32, Boulder, Co.: WICHE, pp. 20–32.

Research Terminology

Knowledge of research language and commonly used terms is necessary to read and understand research. Learning the basic research vocabulary will make your reading of research more meaningful, more enjoyable, and more efficient.

Directions

Define and give an example of the following research terms in the space provided. Consult the Glossary at the end of this book to check the accuracy of your definitions.

Concepts:

Operational definition:

Variable:

Independent variable:

Dependent variable:

Uncontrolled or **extraneous confounding variables:**

Hypotheses:

Data:

Instruments:

Reliability:

Validity:

Population and **sample:**

The Hawthorne effect:

The Halo effect:

Double-blind method:

Audit trail:

Basic social problem:

Basic social process:

Case study:

Confirmability:

Credibility:

Critical social theory:

Data triangulation:

Dependability:

Document analysis:

Ethical inquiry:

Ethnography:

Feminist inquiry:

Field research:

Grounded theory methodology:

Hermeneutics:

Historical method:

Methodological note:

Naturalistic:

Observational note:

Participant observation:

Personal note:

Phenomenology:

Process consenting:

Semistructured interview:

Substantive theory:

Theoretical note:

Transferability:

Unstructured interview:

27 ## Research Symbols

Symbols or abbreviations of research terms are all parts of the research language. The symbols serve to save space.

Directions

Review the end papers of this book. Match the following abbreviations with the terms that they represent. See how many you recognize before resorting to the answers at the back of the book.

Terms	Symbols
_____ 1. Population	β
_____ 2. Linear correlation coefficient	σ
_____ 3. Value of a single score	s
_____ 4. Mean of scores in a sample	μ
_____ 5. Frequency with which a value occurs	$>$
_____ 6. Null hypothesis	s^2
_____ 7. Hypothesis	x
_____ 8. Variance of a set of values	n
_____ 9. Variance of all values in a population	α
_____10. Greater than	$\bar{x}$
_____11. Probability of a type II error	$<$
_____12. Less than	H_1
_____13. Chi-square distribution	N
_____14. Sample	H_0
_____15. Probability of a type I error or the area of the critical region	χ^2
_____16. Standard deviation of all values in a population	f
_____17. Probability	p
_____18. Standard deviation of a set of sample values	r
_____19. Mean of scores in a population	σ^2

Answers to be found at the back of the book.

Learning the Vocabulary of Theory

As you read theories and their relationship to nursing research, you will immediately become aware of the frequent use of some new and esoteric language. An understanding of this vocabulary is essential for you to be able to appreciate and apply the ideas in your reading and in your practice and research.

Directions

Match the terms on the left with the appropriate definitions at the right. Place the correct letter in the spaces provided.

Terms	Definitions
_____ 1. **Theory**	A. This refers to the concepts that structure or offer a framework of propositions for conducting research.
_____ 2. **Conceptual mapping**	
_____ 3. **Conceptual framework**	B. Abstract concepts constructed by the researcher or derived from existing theory.
_____ 4. **Theoretical model**	C. An explanation of the world; a vision or view on truth or reality; a set of interrelated constructs, concepts, and propositions that present a systematic view of phenomena by specifying relationships for the purpose of describing, explaining, and predicting.
_____ 5. **Construct**	
_____ 6. **Proposition**	
_____ 7. **Model**	
_____ 8. **Concept**	D. These are the building blocks of theories and may vary from the empirical to the theoretical.
	E. Several interrelated theories that provide rationale for a research protocol.
	F. These describe the relationships of two or more concepts.
	G. An analogy or symbolic representation of an idea that is revealed in a diagram, picture, or by a mathematical equation.
	H. A kind of theoretical model that aids in the conceptualization of the research problem, or, if you are doing theory generation, the model aids in the visualization of the theory and the interrelationships of the variables.

Answers to be found at the back of the book.

Reference

Kerlinger, N. (1973). *Foundations of Behavioral Research*. New York: Holt, Rinehart & Winston.

Types of Theory

The process of theory building occurs in the mind of the researcher, who has more or less interaction with the empirical world. The degree of involvement with the real world has an influence on the type of theory that is proposed. The three types of theories are *grand theories, middle-range theories,* and *abstracted empiricism.*

Directions

Read the Introduction to this book and definitions of type of theory in the Glossary. Match the descriptive phrases on the right with the types of theory on the left. Place the correct letter in the blank spaces provided under each theory.

Type of Theory

I. **Grand theory**

 — —

 — —

 — —

 — —

II. **Middle-range theory**

 — —

 — —

 — —

 — —

III. **Abstracted empiricism**

 — —

 — —

Descriptive Phrases

A. These theories look at a piece of reality and identify a few key variables.

B. These theories are composed of numerous global concepts that are poorly defined.

C. Propositions are clear in these theories.

D. The scope of the problem in these theories is limited, which encourages in-depth exploration and analysis of a selected topic.

E. The facts in these theories are in isolation from any theory.

F. These theories attempt to explain everything about a subject.

G. The specific focus of these theories is only on empirical phenomena.

H. The focus of these theories is concrete and near-sighted.

I. The constructs and propositions of these theories are nonexistent or are vague and appear to have little basis in the practical world.

J. These are substantive theories, that is, theories about an empirical area (e.g., a psychiatric hospital).

K. Models derived from these theories are either impossible or incomprehensible.

L. The underlying assumption of these theories is that the accumulation of many pieces of data will ultimately and clearly suggest relationships among the data.

M. These theories are not grounded in empirical data.
N. Hypotheses can be derived to test these theories.
O. These theories are not useful as guides for nursing practice.
P. These theories permit suggestions for nursing practice.
Q. Sensitizing concepts can be derived from these theories.
R. To generate these theories, the researcher is close to the empirical world and often uses the methods of field research.
S. These theories propose "irrelevant . . . monolithic concepts" (Mills, 1959, p. 45).
T. These theories fit the empirical world from which they are derived.

Answers to be found at the back of the book.

Reference

Mills, C. W. (1959). *The Sociological Imagination*. New York: Oxford University Press.

Getting to Know Nursing Theorists and Their Grand Theories

30

This exercise will acquaint you with the perspective of some of the major nursing theorists and give you a feeling for the historical development of nursing theory. If the brief synopsis of any theory catches your interest, you can read more about it by going directly to the writings of the particular theorist.

Directions

Match the nursing theorists on the left with the brief synopses of their theories on the right. Place the letter of the synopsis to the left of the nursing theorist.

Nursing Theorist

_____ 1. Florence Nightingale

_____ 2. Lydia Hall

_____ 3. Virginia Henderson

_____ 4. Hildegard Peplau

_____ 5. Faye Abdellah

_____ 6. Dorothea Orem

_____ 7. Martha Rogers

_____ 8. Myra Levine

_____ 9. Sister Calista Roy

_____ 10. Imogene King

_____ 11. Betty Neuman

_____ 12. Rosemary Rizzo Parse

_____ 13. Madeline Leininger

_____ 14. Jean Watson

Theory Synopsis

A. This theorist proposes a health care systems model that views the person as a complete system with parts and subparts that interrelate. People are subject to intrapersonal, interpersonal, and extrapersonal stressors and have flexible lines of resistance that help defend against these stressors.

B. This theorist proposes four conservation principles that aim to alter patients' adaptation processes in positive ways. The four principles include conservation of patient energy, conservation of structural integrity, conservation of personal integrity, and conservation of social integrity.

C. This theorist offers a theory of self-care that centers on the individual. There are six categories of universal self-care requisites, and if the individual cannot meet self-care needs because of illness, injury, or disease, the nurse offers "health deviation self-care."

D. This theorist proposes a general systems theory that includes three dynamic interacting systems: personal systems, interpersonal systems, and social systems.

E. This theorist views "human becoming" as the basis of nursing's uniqueness. Science is viewed as humanistic, rather than mechanistic. People and the environment are two energy fields that are always open, have pattern and organization, and change continuously and creatively.

F.   This theorist's adaptation theory views people as biopsychosocial beings who have to continually adapt to a variety of stimuli, which she calls "focal," "contextual," and "residual." Specific adaptive modes—basic physiological needs, self-concept, role function, and interdependence—help people cope with the changing environment.

G.   This theorist views nursing as a "significant therapeutic interpersonal process." Her theory focuses on the four phases of the nurse–patient relationship: 1) orientation, 2) identification, 3) exploitation, and 4) resolution.

H.   This theorist is noted for her definition of nursing stated in 1955: "Nursing is primarily assisting the individual (sick or well) in the performance of those activities contributing to health or its recovery (or a peaceful death) that s/he would perform unaided if s/he had the necessary strength, will, or knowledge. It is likewise the unique contribution of nursing to help the individual to be independent of such assistance as soon as possible."

I.   This theorist presents the three "aspects of nursing": the person (core of nursing), the disease (cure of nursing), and the body (care of nursing). Her philosophy developed from her work at the Loeb Long-term Care Center in the Bronx. Depending on the patient's problems, each of the three aspects of nursing might be emphasized or de-emphasized.

J.   This theorist classifies nursing problems into 21 categories. She views the nurse as a problem solver whose goal is to identify and then remedy these biopsychosocial problems.

K.   This person was nursing's first nursing theorist. She focused on the physical environment, believing that if nurses altered the environment in a positive fashion, the reparative process could begin.

L.   This theorist views humanity as being dependent upon human caring for its survival. Nursing has historically carried the banner of caring as its core value. While the health care system has not fully recognized caring as a critical element in society's wellness, this theorist cites caring as necessary in developing nursing as a science. She calls nursing interventions, carative factors.

M. This theorist views caring as the core or central focus of nursing. Caring styles and patterns are culturally determined and, therefore, vary transculturally. To be effective caring must be culturally congruent. Contextual factors such as religion, kinship, technology, and education influence patterns of care giving and care seeking.

N. This theorist refers to "cocreation" as an entity that involves unitary man interrelating with the environment. Health is viewed as being cocreated in this process. Her nursing theory of man-living-health is viewed as a continuous process of transcending and reaching beyond the actual.

Answers to be found at the back of the book.

Parts of a Research Article

Most research journal articles are divided into sections with headings and subheadings. If you are aware of the format, you have a better chance of getting your own articles published, and you will be able to read and understand research articles faster because you understand the context.

Directions

Put the following parts of a research article in order of their appearance and give a definition of each. Use major headings. One of the major headings will have two subheadings; one will have four subheadings. Consult the Glossary to check the accuracy of your definitions.

References

Results (conclusions)

Research design

Method

Abstract

Materials needed (data collection)

Statement of study's purpose

Introduction

Discussion/conclusion

Literature review

Procedures (data analysis)

Sample

Answers to be found at the back of the book.

The Scientific Merit of Clinical Nursing Research

32

Nursing practice should be based on sound nursing research rather than on intuition, trial and error, or authority and tradition. As you read nursing journals, you will want to think about which clinical studies have scientific merit and possible utility for your clinical setting.

Directions

Read a clinical research study in one of the nursing research journals that focuses on your area of interest: psychiatry, medical/surgical nursing, or maternal/infant care. Analyze the article based on Fawcett's (1982) list of questions:

1. Was pilot work conducted?
2. If so, are the findings similar?
3. Is corroboration of the findings in clinical situations done with actual patients who receive nursing care?
4. What was the risk or benefit of the nursing action tested in the study?
5. Does the study focus on a significant clinical practice problem?
6. Do nurses have clinical control over study variables?
7. Is it feasible to implement the nursing action in the real world?
8. What is the cost of implementing the nursing action?
9. What contribution to direct health status does the nursing action make?
10. What overall contribution to nursing knowledge does the study make?

Discussion Guidelines

Discuss the following questions in a small group of colleagues or fellow students:

1. Does the author or authors of the article give enough information so you can answer all of Fawcett's questions?
2. If not, for which questions do you require more information?
3. Which of Fawcett's questions are the easiest to answer?

Reference

Fawcett, J. (1982). Utilization of nursing research findings. *Image: Journal of Nursing Scholarship,* June, *14,* 57–59.

Steps in the Research Process

33

The research process is the tool of science by which the goals of science—generating and verifying theories—are realized. The article "Nurse Practitioner Managed Care for Persons with HIV Infection" (Aiken, et al. 1993) illustrates steps in the research process described by Wilson (1993).

Directions

Reread the Introduction to this Part. Find the article in the library and, as you read it, think about how well the author presents each of the following steps in the research process.

Step 1 Stating the research problem

Step 2 Defining the purpose of the research

Step 3 Reviewing related literature to develop a **theoretical framework** and/or place the study in the context of existing knowledge

Step 4 Formulating **hypotheses** and defining **variables**

Step 5 Selecting the **research design**

Step 6 Selecting the **population** and **sample**

Step 7 Conducting a **pilot study**

Step 8 Collecting the **data**

Step 9 Analyzing the data

Step 10 Communicating conclusions

Discussion Guidelines

Discuss the following questions in a group of fellow students or colleagues.

1. Is the research question clearly stated?
2. Does the purpose of the research let the reader know why the question is important? Does it let the reader know what to expect from the study?
3. Are existing theories and concepts, research methods, and findings related to the study question and purpose?
4. Are the hypotheses, if any, stated clearly? Are the concepts or variables clearly and operationally defined so they can be measured?
5. Does the research design clearly delineate how the study will be carried out from data collection through data analysis?
6. Is the sample clearly defined? Is the selected sample a logical choice given the research problem and literature review?
7. If there was a pilot study, did it increase awareness of the strengths and weaknesses of the study's design, sample, and instrument?
8. Are the data collection methods, or instruments, in keeping with the research question and theoretical framework?
9. Are the statistical procedures appropriate for the level and type of data collected? Are the qualitative data methods clearly described?
10. Has the author clearly and logically helped the reader to understand the meaning of the study, its strengths and weaknesses, its implications for practice or education?

11. Has the author made recommendations for further research that evolved from the present study?

References

Aiken, L. et al. (1993). Nurse Practitioner Managed Care for Persons with HIV Infection. *Image: Journal of Nursing Scholarship, 25*(3), 172–177.

Wilson, H. S. (1993). *Introducing Research in Nursing,* 2nd ed. Menlo Park, CA.: Addison-Wesley.

Reading Abstracts

Almost all research journals print abstracts at the beginning of research articles. The purpose of an abstract is to summarize the entire piece as briefly as possible. You will want to read abstracts at an inspectional or analytical level or to decide if you want to read the article at all. Reading abstracts will help save you time.

Directions

Read the following abstracts, and think about the essential information that an abstract should impart: (1) the purpose, objectives, research questions, or **hypotheses**; (2) a description of the **sample**; (3) data collection and analysis procedures; and (4) a summary of important findings. In the space provided after each abstract, write the appropriate information that you found.

Abstract
Title: Comparison of Patient-Controlled and Nurse-Controlled Antiemetic Therapy in Patients Receiving Chemotherapy

The purpose of this quasi-experimental pilot study was to compare the effect of patient-controlled (PCAE) and nurse administered (NCAE) antiemetic therapy for controlling chemotherapy–induced nausea and vomiting in patients receiving moderate emetogenic chemotherapy. Twenty subjects were randomly assigned to either the PCAE group who received IV antiemetic medication via a patient-controlled pump or the NCAE group who received antiemetic medication via nurse administered minibags. Nausea, vomiting, sedation, and drug consumption were measured. There was no difference in nausea scores between the two groups. Subjects in the PCAE group consumed significantly less medication than subjects in the NCAE group.

Source: Edwards, J. N., Herman, J., Wallace, B. K., Pavy, M. D., & Harrison-Pavy, J. (1991). Comparison of patient-controlled and nurse-controlled antiemetic therapy in patients receiving chemotherapy. *Research in Nursing and Health, 14*(3), 249–257.

1. Purpose, objectives, research questions, or hypotheses:

2. Description of the sample:

3. Data collection and analysis procedures:

4. Summary of important findings:

Abstract
Title: Obstetrical Role Strain for Male Nursing Students

The educational experiences of male nursing students are sometimes influenced by the fact that nursing is stereotyped as an occupation for women (Turnipseed, 1986). Because male students are often in the minority, they may experience stress and role strain that can interfere with the achievement of their goals, threaten their self-concept, and affect their success (Flynn & Gooding, 1979; Turnipseed, 1986). The intent of this investigation was to determine if there was a significantly greater reported role strain for male than female baccalaureate nursing students in the obstetrical area.

Source: Sherrod, R. A. (1991). Obstetrical role strain for male nursing students. *Western Journal of Nursing Research,*13(4), 494–502.

1. Purpose, objectives, research questions, or hypotheses:

2. Description of the sample:

3. Data collection and analysis procedures:

4. Summary of important findings:

Abstract
Title: The Healing Process of Female Adult Incest Survivors:
Constructing a Personal Residence

This study generated a descriptive theoretical framework of the healing process of adult survivors of incest based on the perceptions of 11 survivors who had experienced some degree of healing. The core variable that emerged from the data was labeled "constructing personal residence" to reflect the participants' descriptions of their experiences as laborious, active, and constructive. The process of constructing a residence included three main elements: building a new relationship with the self, regulating one's relationship with others, and influencing the community in a meaningful way.

Source: Draucker, C. B. (1991). The healing process of female adult incest survivors: Constructing a personal residence. *Image: Journal of Nursing Scholarship, 24*(1), 4–8.

1. Purpose, objectives, research questions, or hypotheses:

2. Description of the sample:

3. Data collection and analysis procedures:

4. Summary of important findings:

Discussion Guidelines

Discuss the following questions with colleagues or fellow students:

1. Are any of the abstracts incomplete in any of the four parts?
2. Are the abstracts clear?
3. Are they organized in a logical fashion that mirrors the research process?

Reference

Wilson, H. S. (1993). *Introducing research in nursing.* (2e) Menlo Park, CA: Addison-Wesley.

35 Categories of Research Questions in Nursing

Most types of research questions in nursing fall into the categories of (a) **factor-isolating** or "naming" questions; (b) **factor-relating** questions that ask "What is happening?"; (c) **situation-relating** questions that ask "What will happen if?"; and (d) **situation-producing** questions that ask "How can I make it happen?" Understanding which type of question guides a study enables the reader to anticipate the level of the study.

Directions

Each of the following research questions is an example of one of the four categories just listed. Indicate the type of research question by putting the appropriate letter in the space provided at the left.

Type of Research Question

A. Factor-isolating
B. Factor-relating
C. Situation-relating
D. Situation-producing

Research Question

_____ 1. What is the relation between hope and remission in cancer patients?

_____ 2. What are the contexts in which nurse–physician arguments occur?

_____ 3. How does humor affect patients with chronic pain?

_____ 4. What are the factors that help diabetic patients to learn self-care?

_____ 5. What are the stages in the recovering process of alcoholism?

_____ 6. Will patient education increase compliance in a cardiac rehabilitation program?

_____ 7. What are the consequences for nurses who have been sued in malpractice suits?

_____ 8. Will positive reinforcement decrease acting-out behavior among acting-out adolescents?

_____ 9. What is the relation between birth control pills and thrombophlebitis in women under 30 years of age?

_____10. How can nursing interventions promote patient compliance?

_____11. Will relaxation exercises increase the feeling of well-being of patients in nursing homes?

_____12. How can nurses intervene to prevent combative behavior among psychiatric patients?

_____13. What is the relationship between nurses' education and their concern for patients' social–psychological needs?

_____14. Will egg crate mattresses decrease the number of decubiti on quadriplegic patients?

_____15. What is the relationship between the presence of a significant other during a woman's labor and the woman's perception of her labor?

_____16. How can team nursing encourage feelings of positive regard among nurses?

Answers to be found at the back of the book.

36 Understanding the Purpose of Specific Study Designs

Each study design has a general purpose. It is most important that you understand the purpose of different study designs so that you can accurately critique the types of designs used (i.e., do they allow the study's purpose to be met?), and so you will be able to choose an appropriate design for your own research.

Directions

Use the Glossary at the back of the book to look up the definitions for types of study designs. Match the type of study design with the appropriate purpose. Put the corresponding letter in the space provided at the left.

Type of Study Design

_____ 1. **Historical study design**

_____ 2. **Case study design**

_____ 3. **Survey research design**

_____ 4. **Experimental study design**

_____ 5. **Quasi-experimental design**

_____ 6. **Ex post facto study design**

_____ 7. **Methodological studies**

_____ 8. **Grounded theory study design**

_____ 9. **Phenomenology study design**

_____10. **Ethnographic study design**

_____11. **Hermeneutics study design**

Purpose of Study Design

A. To describe characteristics, opinions, attitudes, or behaviors as they currently exist in a population

B. To manipulate and control one or more independent variables and observe the dependent variable or variables for the consequences, change, outcome, or effect

C. To study something after the fact; that is, subjects who have undergone some life experiences

D. To explain the present or to anticipate the future based on a systematic collection and critical evaluation of data pertaining to past occurrences

E. To provide an in-depth analysis of a subject for investigation, such as an individual patient, a family, a hospital ward, a health-care agency, or a professional organization or group

F. To use an alternative design similar to an experimental design when random assignment to control and experimental groups cannot be implemented. For example, the nonequivalent pretest-posttest control group design

G. To develop tools or instruments that are suited to answering nursing questions

H. To describe the lived experience by using examplars, paradigm cases, and constitutive patterns
I. To study a culture or subculture
J. To generate a substantive theory about an empirical area of inquiry
K. To describe in detail the lived experience

Answers to be found at the back of the book.

37 Matching Research Designs and Research Purpose

Every research design has its own specific purpose. Diers (1979) grouped research purposes into four categories: factor-naming, factor-relating, association-testing, and causal hypothesis-testing studies. The research design must allow the researcher to meet the purpose of the research.

Directions

Match each of the following research designs with the correct research purpose. Put the letter of the research purpose in the space provided at the left. Note that the designs may have more than one purpose.

Research Design

_____ 1. Historical study designs

_____ 2. Case study designs

_____ 3. Survey research designs

_____ 4. Experimental study designs

_____ 5. Quasi-experimental designs

_____ 6. Ex post facto study designs

Answers to be found at back of book.

Research Purpose

A. Factor-naming

B. Factor-relating

C. Association-testing (correlational)

D. Causal hypothesis-testing studies

Discussion Guidelines

Discuss your answers with colleagues or fellow students. If you have any questions about the answers, refer to Wilson's *Introducing Research in Nursing* 2e (1993).

References

Diers, D. (1979). *Research in Nursing Practice*. Philadelphia: Lippincott.

Wilson, H. S. (1993). *Introducing Research in Nursing.* (2e) Menlo Park, CA: Addison-Wesley.

Recognizing Research Designs*

> Every study has its own specific purpose. Certain research designs are more or less useful in helping the researcher achieve the research objectives.

Directions

Indicate the research design that correctly identifies the following examples. Write the corresponding letter of the research design in the space provided.

    A. Descriptive/observational research

    B. Correlational research

    C. Experimental research

    D. Quasi-experimental research

_____ 1. A researcher is interested in astrological differences in extroversion and hypothesizes that people of certain astrological signs are more extroverted than others. An extroversion score is obtained from 120 subjects–10 from each of the 12 signs. These extroversion scores are later compared.

_____ 2. A researcher is interested in "discussion" versus "lecture" approaches to nurse training and believes that the former is better. At a large hospital, half the wards are randomly designated to receive the discussion approach, the other half to receive lectures. Later, performance on a nursing mastery index is recorded for each nurse and then compared by group.

_____ 3. A researcher is interested in the weight-loss behaviors of people diagnosed with anorexia nervosa and/or bulimia. Patients of both types are given a questionnaire that categorizes several weight-loss techniques (fasting, vomiting, laxatives, etc.). The number of patients utilizing each technique is tabulated.

_____ 4. A researcher is interested in demonstrating a positive relation between caffeine intake and blood pressure. Patients in a stress clinic are asked how many drinks containing caffeine they consume daily, and each patient's blood pressure is recorded.

_____ 5. A researcher is interested in demonstrating that emergency room nurses undergo more stress than nurses in intensive care units. Several stress indices are recorded from nurses in both environments. These stress scores are then compared.

_____ 6. A researcher is interested in the "frustration-aggression" hypothesis. At random, half the subjects are told they failed a research methods test ("high frustration" group), while the other half are told they passed ("low frustration"

*SOURCE: R. Powell, PhD, University of North Florida.

group). In the guise of another study, subjects are then asked to pick five of their favorite TV shows. The number of violent TV shows chosen by each subject is recorded and later compared by group.

_____ 7. Another researcher is interested in the "frustration-aggression" hypothesis. A standardized personality test is administered, which yields a "frustration predisposition" and an "aggression tendency" score for each subject. The relationship between these scores is then ascertained.

Answers to be found at the back of the book.

Discussion Guidelines

If you have any questions regarding the correct answers, discuss them with your fellow students or colleagues. Or, consult a text on research designs or Wilson's *Introducing Research in Nursing* (1993).

Reference

Wilson, H. S. (1993). *Introducing Research in Nursing.* (2e) Menlo Park, CA: Addison-Wesley.

Elements of Research Designs

Research designs have certain elements: **Setting, subjects, sample**, procedure for protection of subjects, instrumentation (if appropriate), procedure for data collection, procedure for data analysis. Each element should be described in detail for each research study.

Directions

Fill in the blanks with the element that correctly completes each of the following statements.

1. _____ refers to process of informing research participants about the risk/benefits of the research and their rights as participants.
2. _____ is where the research will take place.
3. _____ will be the recipients of the experimental treatment in an experimental design or the participants in a nonexperimental design.
4. _____ refers to a reasonable number of subjects/participants so that the researcher can make comparisons or describe a phenomenon and the procedure for obtaining them.
5. _____ refers to specific strategies to obtain data, and types of data.
6. _____ refers to plans for analyzing/interpreting the data.
7. _____ refers to tools, for example, questionnaires, measuring devices used to collect data.

Answers to be found at the back of the book.

40 **Searching Out Elements of Research Designs in Published Research**

We assume that the six generic elements are vital to all types of research designs. If the elements are not described, the reader is left with unanswered questions and a lack of clarity about the design.

Directions

Choose articles from nursing research journals and try to identify the six generic elements by answering the following questions (note the suggested references at the end of this exercise).

1. What is the **setting**?
2. Who are the **subjects**?
3. How many people, records, and so on comprise the **sample**, and how are they obtained?
4. What is the **treatment** (if **experimental design**), or what are the conditions under which **data** will be collected (if **nonexperimental design**)?
5. What are the measurement, observation, or data-collection methods?
6. How are the data analyzed and interpreted?

Discussion Guidelines

Discuss the following questions with fellow students or colleagues.

1. If any of the studies was missing one or more of the elements, what was the effect of the omission on the logic and coherence of the study?
2. Does the omission of any one of the elements appear to be more vital than that of any other element? Or do you think each element is equally important?

References

Abraham, I., Neundorfer, M., & Currie, L. J. (1992). Effects of group interventions on cognition and depression in nursing home residents. *Nursing Research, 41*(4), 196–202.

DeMonterice, D., Meier, P. P., Engstrom, J. L., Crichton, C. L., & Mangurten, H. H. (1992). Concurrent validity of a new instrument for measuring nutritive sucking in preterm infants. *Nursing Research, 41*(6), 342–346.

Gift, A. G., Moore, T., & Soeken, K. (1992). Relaxation to reduce dyspnea and anxiety in COPD patients. *Nursing Research, 41*(4), 242–246.

Hartweg, D. L. (1993). Self-care actions of healthy middle-age women to promote well-being. *Nursing Research, 42*(4), 221–227.

41 Categorizing Sources of Error in Research

In good research, a **study design** must be matched to the tasks of answering the specified study questions and to controlling **extraneous variables** that could detract from the value of study findings. This exercise will familiarize you with sources of **error** in research.

Directions

The three major categories of sources or error in research are listed on the left. Examples of each category are listed on the right. Match the examples on the right to the major categories on the left. Put the corresponding number in the space provided at the left.

Categories of Sources of Error

I. Inadequate and inaccurate data
    - _____A.
    - _____B.
    - _____C.
    - _____D.
    - _____E.

II. Mechanical errors
    - _____A.
    - _____B.
    - _____C.

III. Fallacies in interpretation
    - _____A.
    - _____B.
    - _____C.
    - _____D.
    - _____E.
    - _____F.

Examples

1. Mistakes in arithmetic and other mathematical processes
2. Unrepresentative samples
3. Unreliable standards and units of measurement
4. Ignoring negative evidence
5. Application of wrong formulas
6. Inaccurate data resulting from poor observation and carelessness
7. Mistaking correlation for causation
8. Errors in copying
9. Comparing noncomparable data
10. Insufficient data
11. Generalizing from too few cases
12. Distorting interpretations to fit preconceptions and prejudices
13. Deliberately falsified data
14. Failing to consider all significant factors

Answers to be found at the back of the book.

42 Evaluation of Abstract and Title for Research Proposals

Most proposals begin with an **abstract**, the purpose of which is to convey the essence of the proposed study to the reviewers. The abstract presents the central idea of the study and convinces the reader that it is both interesting and important. The title serves similar purposes, but in an even more abbreviated way, using key terms that *make sense* and orient the reader to the nature of the study.

Directions

Read the following abstracts and titles from nursing research proposals.

Abstracts

Title: An Observational Study of Alzheimer's Dementia (AD) Behavioral Symptoms

Principal Investigator: Sally Hutchinson, RN, PhD, FAAN

Consultant: Holly S. Wilson, RN, PhD, FAAN

This application is for funding to conduct a rigorous observational study for the purpose of describing and categorizing the full range of behavioral symptoms among diagnosed AD patients in a specialized AD day-care program. The goal of this research is to generate basic knowledge for the long range objective of developing a controlled clinical trial of nursing interventions to manage symptoms and preserve functioning in AD patients. Specific aims are to use observational methodology, videotape technology, and the analytic methods of qualitative ethology to: 1) generate rich descriptive detail about the range of variation and the patterns of behavioral symptoms of AD and 2) describe and explain environmental and interactional contextual conditions associated with AD symptom variations and patterns. The setting for this research is a specialized AD day-care center. After consent is obtained data collection will involve videotaping a minimum of 50 patients engaged in the following activities: 1) hygiene and grooming, 2) dressing, 3) eating, 4) toileting, 5) structured activities, 6) unstructured activities, and 7) social interactions. The video-camera is equipped with a microphone to allow the researcher to dictate ongoing field observations. A minimum of 150 hours of videotaped observations will be obtained over the three-year study period. Ongoing descriptive data about the patients will be maintained. The outcome of data analysis will be a classification (taxonomy) of the kinds of AD behavioral symptoms and rich, detailed descriptions (ethogram) of the range and patterns of AD behavioral symptoms as they occur in their interactional and environmental contexts. Once this groundwork is completed, delineation of appropriate nursing interventions for an individual symptom or a cluster of symptoms can be accomplished.

Source: Academic Research Enhancement Award. Awarded by the National Institute of Nursing Research. Reference Number R15NR03366, 1993.

Title: The Use of Adjunctive Music Auditory Therapy to Reduce Chronic Cancer Pain Intensity

Author: Lucile R. Cuenot

Provision of pain relief has been identified as a primary research priority in oncology today. Clients with chronic cancer pain due to metastatic progression have been victims of a multidimensional problem for many years, yet there has been limited research on the use of adjunctive auditory distraction therapies. The purpose of this quasi-experimental research is to determine if chronic cancer pain intensity will be reduced with music as an adjunctive auditory distraction therapy among clients on routine pharmacologic pain management regimens. The research hypothesis under investigation is the following: Chronic cancer pain clients who listen to self-selected music recordings will report a greater reduction in pain intensity than clients who have no adjunctive music auditory distraction therapy.

A list of chronic cancer pain clients being hospitalized will be obtained from the participating oncologists at each facility on a weekly basis. After a full explanation of the purpose and procedures within the study, each client who desires to participate will sign a consent form. Demographic data will be collected on a convenience sample of forty clients. The clients will be randomly assigned to two groups, one that listens to self-selected music and one that does not. The music group will also answer a modified Hartsock Music Preference Questionnaire to determine musical preferences and lengths of listening times for comparisons. Pain intensity, the dependent variable, for each client will be measured by a visual-analog scale (VAS) before and after a 45-minute interval. The comparison group will be encouraged to assume a position of comfort within their hospital room and be advised to continue whatever activities they choose to manage their pain—as long as the activity does not involve listening to music. Subjects will be given the suggestion that this period of time will allow for their management of pain intensity in whatever way they consider best.

A repeated measures analysis of variance will be employed to determine the difference in pain intensity reduction between and among the two groups. Demographic information will provide descriptive variables to further describe the sample.

The significance of this study to nursing is to provide additional support for the use of distraction theory within the clinical management of chronic cancer pain when optimal medication regimens are not fully effective. By providing additional data to support the gate control theory of pain, and increasing the knowledge and application of auditory distraction therapies to clinical practice, more creative nursing interventions can be used to manage the multidimensional problem of chronic cancer pain.

Source: Unpublished master thesis. (1993). University of Florida College of Nursing.

Title: Animal Assisted Therapy with Hospitalized Adolescents

Author: Norine Bardill

Adolescents with acute and chronic psychiatric problems experience multiple losses. Research shows the human/companion animal bond has the potential to improve the quality of life for people dealing with losses. The purpose of this descriptive study is to describe the responses of hospitalized adolescents to a cocker spaniel who resides on a sixteen-bed hospital psychiatric unit. Data collection includes patient journals, observations, and interviews with ten patients. The ethnographic method will be used for data analysis.
Source: Unpublished master thesis. (1994). University of Florida College of Nursing.

Title: Differences in Maternal Perceptions of Childbirth With or Without Epidural Anesthesia

Author: Lisa P. Malecki

The purpose of this descriptive research is to determine if there is a difference in maternal perception of childbirth with or without epidural anesthesia. Mercer's role attainment theory, which proposes that maternal perceptions of childbirth potentially affect self-esteem and mothering behaviors, and thus, maternal role attainment, is used as the theoretical rationale. Sixty subjects having a vaginal delivery of a normal newborn will be placed in either the epidural or nonepidural group. The Attitudes about the Labor and Delivery Experience questionnaire will be administered within the first 48 hours postpartum. The data will be analyzed with independent sample t-tests and chi-square procedures. The findings may help nurses counsel women about pain relief options in labor.

Source: Unpublished master thesis. (1993). University of Florida College of Nursing.

Discussion Guidelines

Discuss the following questions with a group of fellow students or colleagues.

1. Is the abstract within the 300-word limit?
2. Is the abstract clear?
3. Does it cover the important points?
4. Does it present central ideas?
5. Are you convinced of the study's importance?
6. Does the title make sense?
7. Does the title fit with the abstract?

Evaluating the Problem Statement in Research Proposals

The statement of the research problem usually introduces a proposal. It must convince reviewers that the proposed study is important, and it should reduce the scope of the problem to manageable terms by specifying a study focus. Funding decisions are influenced by the clarity with which an investigator conveys how a particular piece of research will contribute to the theory or overall knowledge of general or specific phenomena. For the purpose of this exercise, you will be a member of a peer review group who evaluates research proposals.

Directions

Read the following examples of statements of nursing problems.

Problem Statement

Title: The Process of Developing Personal Sovereignty in Women Who Repeatedly Acquire Sexually Transmitted Diseases

Authors: Nancy Redfern, RN, CNM, MN, Sally Hutchinson, RN, PhD, FAAN

Research Problem

"In the time it takes to read this sentence, a man or woman between the ages of fifteen and thirty will get a sexually transmitted disease" (STD) (Davis, 1988, p. 25). Sexually transmitted diseases continue to escalate as a public health menace according to the Centers for Disease Control (CDC). CDC researchers report 4 million new cases of chlamydia, 2 million of gonorrhea, 100,000 of syphilis, and 500,000 to 1 million new cases of pelvic inflammatory disease each year in the United States. Goldsmith (1989) notes there are currently 12 million cases of genital warts with 750,000 new cases per year, and 20–30 million cases of genital herpes with 500,000 new cases per year. STDs with open lesions make women more susceptible to AIDS. Women comprise the fastest growing category of the AIDS epidemic, accounting for 11.5% of new cases being reported in the United States (Smeltzer & Whipple, 1991). By the year 2000 more women than men are expected to have AIDS (Haines, 1991). Nurses and nurse practitioners see women daily who put their health at risk and pay a high price for their sexual relationships. STDs will cost some of them their lives. Others will suffer ectopic pregnancies or impaired fertility with fallopian tube inflammation and scarring. Many will develop cervical neoplasia as a direct result of human papillovirus. Still others will transmit syphilis or AIDS perinatally to their infants. Treatment is costly for both acute and long-term symptoms.

Many women presenting for STD treatment experience repeat infections. In one inner-city STD clinic, 85% of the 116 female clients had a history of prior STDs, and 52% reported more than one prior episode (Horn et al., 1990). In 1990, the STD branch of the National Institute of Allergy and Infectious Diseases (NIAID) developed an agenda for integrated behavioral research for prevention and control of sexually transmitted diseases. They emphasized the need for qualitative studies to enrich understanding of the social context and the meaning of poorly understood sexual risk-taking behavior (Aral et al., 1990).

The purpose of this grounded theory study is to explore and describe the experiences and perceptions of women who repeatedly acquire STDs, excluding AIDS. By understanding the meanings attached to the woman's experience, interventions may be more effective and acceptable to women at risk. Only when interventions are personally relevant can they be successful.

Source: *Qualitative Health Research*, 1995. Vol 5. pp. 222–236.

Problem Statement

Title: Differences in Maternal Perceptions of Childbirth With or Without Epidural Anesthesia

Author: Lisa Malecki, RN, CNM

Research Problem

Women in today's society may have the option of deciding how to manage the pain of labor. Epidural anesthesia offers a tempting solution. It is considered safe and effective, and offers pain relief during labor and delivery (Taylor, 1985). Epidural anesthesia allows the woman to participate, allows immediate interaction with the newborn by decreasing pain. It also prevents the physiologic sequelae of unrelieved pain in labor that can cause maternal and fetal acidosis, and decreased uteroplacental blood flow (Marrone et al., 1988; Taylor, 1985). It is understandable why some women choose epidural anesthesia over the options of systemic and/or local medications, or no medication at all. However, some researchers suggest that women have a more positive perception of the childbirth experience when they do not have epidural anesthesia (Mercer et al., 1983; Slavazza et al., 1985; Mercer et al., 1985). This is possibly due to an increase in feelings of control and active participation in the childbirth process.

Perception of the childbirth experience is important because it may affect maternal-newborn interaction and maternal role attainment (Mercer, 1981). Maternal role attainment is a complex social and cognitive process that is learned rather than intuitive (Rubin, 1967). A basic assumption of maternal role attainment theory is that a woman defines her performance in a role and responds according to her perceptions of past and present experiences (Mercer, 1983). Further research is needed to determine whether epidural anesthesia affects the maternal perception of childbirth. This research will attempt to answer the question: What is the difference in maternal perceptions of childbirth with or without epidural anesthesia?

Source: unpublished masters' thesis. (1993). University of Florida College of Nursing.

Discussion Guidelines

Discuss the following questions with fellow students or colleagues.

1. Is the problem stated with precision?
2. Does the problem merit study?
3. Is there a possible solution to the problem?
4. Is the problem intelligible to a reader who is generally sophisticated but who may be relatively uninformed in the specific area of investigation?
5. Does the problem suggest the significance of conducting the study?

44 ## Evaluating the Review of Related Literature in a Research Proposal

Nursing research that is designed to solve practical clinical problems and studies that are conducted to test or yield knowledge for knowledge's sake must be placed in the context of what scientific work has gone before.

Directions

Read the following literature review.

Literature Review

Title: An Observational Study of Alzheimers Dementia (AD) Behavioral Symptoms

Principal Investigator: Sally A. Hutchinson, RN, PhD, FAAN
Consultant: Holly S. Wilson, RN, PhD, FAAN

Specific Aims

Professional caregivers suggest that serious problems for AD patients result from their behavioral symptoms such as wandering, incontinence, sleep disturbances, catastrophic outbursts, and the like (Norbeck, J., Chafetz, L., Wilson, H., & Weiss, S., 1991). AD patients often wander into unsafe areas, handle unsafe objects, disassemble objects (exposing hazardous parts), or try to ingest inedible objects. These safety problems also raise significant issues of facility liability (Coons, 1988; Dawson & Reid, 1987; 1985, 1986; Hussian & Davis, 1985). "Nuisance problems" for institutional caregivers occur when patients rummage through the personal possessions of other patients, get into storage areas, walk away with nursing records, and get into the bed of another resident—often with the resident in it (Coon, 1988; Dawson & Reid, 1987; Hiatt, 1985; Rader, 1987). These symptoms not only contribute to decisions to institutionalize affected individuals but also lead to the use of chemical and physical restraints in the institutional setting. While clinical and anecdotal information about intervention methods exists, few controlled clinical trials are available. In this proposed study we will systematically observe, classify, and describe the full range of symptom variations and patterns in a specialized AD day-care center as a basic and preliminary step toward controlled clinical trials of symptom management strategies. Placing symptoms in interpersonal and environmental context is more likely to yield approaches that are effective. Examination of symptoms using checklists fails to capture the relationship of the symptom to the environmental context. In our pilot study (Lucero, Hutchinson, Leger-Krall, & Wilson, 1993) we noticed that wandering on some occasions appeared to be a search for hydration because the patient repeatedly picked up cups from the trash and attempted to drink from them. Our observation of the context revealed that the patient had not had fluids for several hours. Staff documented this behavior merely as "self-stimulatory wandering." Placing the behavior in context in this instance indicated that offering fluids was the appropriate intervention for behavior initially assessed as "wandering." The overall purpose of this application for funding is to conduct a preliminary observational study that will lead to subsequent controlled clinical trials of nonpharmacological management of behavioral symptoms exhibited by AD patients. Specific aims of this proposed study are to: 1) generate rich, descriptive detail about the range of variation and the patterns of AD behavioral symptoms and 2) describe and explain environmental and interactional contextual conditions associated with AD symptom variations and patterns. Once we lay this groundwork, delineation of appropriate nursing interventions for an individual symptom or a cluster of symptoms can be accomplished and tested.

Background and Significance

Alzheimer's disease (AD) is an Organic Mental Disorder associated with critical neurologic degeneration that ravages the minds and robs the personalities of about 4 million Americans (National Institute on Aging, 1990). The incidence of AD in people at 65 years is at least 5–7% and up to 20% in the over 80 age group (Daniels & Irwin, 1989). Half of elders over 85 years (the fastest growing segment of the population) have AD (Health Policy & Biomedical Research of the Week, 1990). AD not only steals a person's mind, but also destroys one's sense of self by progressively undermining one's ability to remember, to reason, even to recognize one's own loved ones.

Advances in Knowledge

Recent research on AD has concentrated for the most part on finding a cause or an accurate biological marker for diagnosing the disorder (Buckwalter, 1989). Issues related to the burdens of family caregiving are receiving increased research attention (Daniels & Irwin, 1980; Gwyther & George, 1986; Fitting, Rabins, Lucas, & Eastham, 1986). Cognitive deficits such as the loss of the intellectual abilities of memory, judgment, abstract thought and other higher cortical functions and associated psychiatric symptomatology (including depression and hallucinations) have captured the interest of some investigators and clinicians. Studies of the last several years have contributed increasing precision to a preliminary descriptive profile of the natural comprehensive profiles to date that clinically differentiate global stages ranging from normal CNS aging to severe AD. Little scientific work, however, has focused on noncognitive behavioral symptoms that are cited by family and professional caregivers as posing the most difficult management problems, and which predominate in the moderate and severe stages.

The Priority of Symptom Management Research

While it is not yet possible to prevent, permanently alter the course, or cure AD, increasing attention is being directed to research that is necessary to develop and test interventions and management strategies that can reduce or help to manage the patient's secondary behavioral symptoms and preserve, to the degree possible, the ability to function in activities of daily living. Some of this research has addressed psychiatric and cognitive symptoms (Merriam et al., 1989) in an attempt to ascertain the prevalence of complaints of affective symptoms like depression and psychotic phenomena such as hallucinations and delusions among AD patients. Findings from such studies have yielded important clinical implications for the appropriateness of pharmacologic treatment of such superimposed treatable psychiatric symptoms. Other studies have focused on assessment of cognitive decline, general confusion, and mental status in AD patients and generated the standardized dementia instruments available in both clinical practice and research. But secondary behavioral symptomatology in AD is only beginning to receive investigative attention. Even fewer studies have addressed treatment of these symptoms and those that do rely primarily on pharmacotherapeutic agents (Martin, 1989). While the recent literature abounds with clinical articles on secondary AD symptoms and associated management problems including thirst, erectile problems, hearing impairment, wandering, sleep activity cycle disturbance, incontinence, and the like, a 1991 MEDLINE search of over 3,000 English citations from 1980–1986 revealed only one study that involved direct observation of selected secondary behavioral symptoms (functional performance in common activities of daily living) in Alzheimer's patients (Skurla, Rogers, & Sunderland, 1988). This study asked 9 AD patients to complete 4 experimental tasks in a laboratory-like setting (the ADL Situation Test) and then examined the relationship of their performance on these daily living tasks to the severity of their dementia noting that severity of dementia was related to increased time in performance of the tasks and decreased task performance. The researcher argued **the value of direct observation** rather than asking caregivers about patients' functional capacities. Most investigators, by contrast, have relied heavily on self or caregiver reports of functional capacity and other behavioral symptoms or the administration of proxy measures in the form of standardized tests and checklists. Many of the studies using instruments such as the Behavioral Problems Checklist (BPC) in a 1988 study of behavioral disturbance and cognitive dysfunction, acknowledge that, "No one measure adequately surveys the range of behavioral problems . . . therefore the checklist was adapted from another behavioral rating scale that used ratings by caregivers in a mixed population of dependent elderly" (Teri et al., 1988, p. 111). These investigators acknowledge further that, "Despite the consistency of opinion regarding the pervasiveness and destructiveness of behavioral problems in AD, there are surprisingly little empirical data on the nature and prevalence of behavioral problems in AD patients" (Teri et al. 1988, p. 1). The validity of self-report measures in institutionalized middle- and late-stage AD subjects is questionable since they may be unreliable or incapable informants. Caregiver reports may also be biased because they depend on caregiver perception and interpretation of the meaning of various behaviors. Two additional studies involving direct observation of self-care capacity were reported in the literature, but one was a case study and the second included subjects with multiple medical conditions and physical impairments that could have influenced behavior. No studies using direct observation to investigate the full range of variation and patterns of secondary behavioral AD symptoms under natural environmental conditions were found in this literature review. The proposed study fills this gap.

Source: Academic Research Enhancement Award. Funded by the National Institute of Nursing Research. Reference Number R15NR03366.

Discussion Guidelines

Discuss the following questions with your colleagues or fellow students.

1. Does the literature review clearly present the theoretical basis, rationale, framework or organizing schema of which the proposed study is a part?
2. Does the review present a mere bibliography or does it analyze or critically appraise the important and recent substantive and methodological developments, and does it indicate how the study adds to what is now known?
3. Does the review support the assumptions, operational definitions, and methodological procedures by showing that the proposed study has, in fact, profited from scholarly and scientific work that has preceded it?

45 Evaluating the Design, Methods, and Procedure Section in Research Proposals

The **design**, **methods**, and **procedure** section of research proposals should tell the readers the activities that will be conducted to accomplish the study objectives or test the study **hypotheses**.

Directions

Read the following design, methods, and procedure sections from nursing research proposals.

Method

Title: An Observational Study of Alzheimer's Dementia (AD) Behavioral Symptoms

Principal Investigator: Sally A. Hutchinson, RN, PhD, FAAN
Consultant: Holly S. Wilson, RN, PhD, FAAN

Method

This observational study design (qualitative ethology) employs video and audiotaping technology to gather the full range of variation and patterns of AD behavioral symptoms under natural conditions in a specialized AD day-care program. This method of systematic direct observation is particularly useful for the study of patients who cannot be interviewed due to conditions such as AD. Our goal in this preliminary study, is to generate an AD behavioral symptom taxonomy as well as to provide a rich textual narrative ethogram that places behaviors in context. We ultimately intend to both portray the descriptive nature of behavioral problems and to seek **conceptual generalizability**. The analysis of patient behaviors in context is a first step. The analysis of nurse behaviors/interventions will follow in a future study.

The Setting

This research will be conducted in a purposively selected specialized AD day-care center in the Southeastern U.S. The setting was selected because: (1) patients admitted to the program have received a clinical diagnosis of probable AD; (2) the program has a capacity of 30 patients/day with an average daily census of 21, assuring the likelihood of capturing a wide range of individual behavioral variation as well as shared patterns; (3) patients are predominantly in the middle stages of dementia wherein they present the most difficult and wide-ranging problematic behavioral symptoms yet patients with early and late stage AD also attend the program; (4) the demographic characteristics of patients provide for the inclusion of women (66%) and minorities (36.36%); (5) the agency endorses this study.

The Sampling Plan and Data Collection

Informed consent will be obtained from authorized family members and staff, since staff are likely to be videotaped as they interact with patients. The sample consists of *behavioral observations* rather than individual subjects. We will observe behavior under natural conditions as it occurs in a minimum of 50 patients during (1) hygiene and grooming, (2) dressing, (3) eating, (4) toileting, (5) structured activities, (6) unstructured activities, (7) social interactions, and (8) arrival and departure from the center. The initial sampling strategy is termed Focal-Subject Sampling. It provides the most rigorous and complete record of a groups' behaviors (Morse & Bottorff, 1990). A focus refers to a single behavioral symptom (e.g., wandering) or a few behavioral symptoms (e.g., wandering, disrobing) and the relationships of such symptoms to the context. We will conduct 3 types of focused observations: (1) focal subject sampling in which we will capture as much variation in behavioral symptoms as is evidenced by the patient population, (2) all event sampling in which we record behavioral symptoms related to a specific event such as eating etc., and (3) sequence sampling in which a chain or sequence of behavior in the order of occurrence is followed by the video camera. When using this strategy as many as possible of the different behavioral elements of the entire patient group are recorded during the typical daily events. In addition to focal sampling, theoretical sampling will be employed during the 3-year data collection period. Relevant observations are those that permit generating, delimiting, and saturating the taxonomy of behavioral symptoms. Saturating the categories of the taxonomy refers to their completeness. Theoretical sampling allows the significant variables to become apparent through the expansion and elaboration of the developing categories. Given the budget constraints, we anticipate a minimum of *150 total observational hours* over 3 years. In the 01 year, videotaped observations for 2 hours will occur 3 times per month from month 04 to month 12 (54 hours). In the 02 year, videotaped observations for 2 hours will occur 2 times per month from month 01 to month 12 (48 hours). In the 03 year, videotaped observations for 2 hours will again occur 3 times per month from month 01 to month 09 (54 hours). Based on pilot research that used videotaped observation and consultation with experts (Morse, personal communication, 1992; Jordan, personal communication, 1992), the weight of this amount of data should be highly appropriate to address the study aims and yet be manageable and feasible for analysis.

Preparing Data for Analysis

Stage 1: Videotapes will be numbered and labeled. "Real-time" will be imprinted on the tapes so that we may locate events and behavioral elements.

Stage 2: We will establish a log to serve as an index to events and behavioral elements located on the tapes. This log is simply a list of events and behavioral elements along with the videotape number, date, time, and brief researcher comments (Morse, 1992). The narratives that place the videotaped behaviors in their interpersonal and environmental context will be transcribed into text using MARTIN, a qualitative software program. This is essential since it is assumed that interactions and the environment influence AD symptoms.

Data Analysis

Initially the transcribed recordings of the videotapes will be discussed with the consultant and the RA. Differences in perception will be resolved by the analytic team as an ongoing process. Data analysis and data collection will go on concurrently. We will use Spradley's (1980) method for making a Taxonomic Analysis. A taxonomy is a set of categories organized on the basis of a single semantic relationship. A taxonomy can reveal subsets of behaviors and the way they are related to the whole on different levels of abstraction (Spradley, 1980). The specific steps for data analysis follow:

Stage 1: Creating a Classification of Behavioral Symptoms (Taxonomy) Step 1. Select the domain for taxonomic analysis. In this case the domain has been predetermined as types of secondary behavioral symptoms of AD. This analytic process begins with playing and replaying the tapes in order to identify and code behavioral elements of interest that will be entered into the log, e.g., wandering. This rich, textual description of behavior will record sufficient detail to represent the behavior itself and initially will avoid interpreting the function or purpose the behavior serves. For example labels such as "anxious," or "withdrawn" will be avoided. Instead we will describe "hand-wringing," "pacing" etc., so that no data are lost due to premature categorization. We will use Rosenblum's guidelines for determining the boundaries for behavioral elements, which are: marked changes in a behavior pattern and shifts in the orientation of the subjects' attention. If a behavioral element is added to the basic pattern being observed, the combined behaviors will be recorded as a separate specific pattern (e.g., "dozing while eating") (Rosenblum, 1978).

Step 2. Look for similarities in the behavioral elements in Step 1 in order to group them into categories. Here we'll ask, "How is wandering during lunch similar to and different to wandering during unstructured time?"

Step 3. Look for additional kinds of wandering by asking of the data, "What are all the kinds of wandering?" and "What are their attributes?" This will allow us to identify the patterns as well as the full range of wandering and other behavioral symptoms in AD patients.

Step 4. Construct a tentative taxonomy. This can be done by creating a box diagram, a figure of lines and nodes or outlining the specific behaviors and the types of behaviors (categories).

Stage 2: Creating a Comprehensive, Textual Analytic Description of Behavioral Symptoms in Context (Ethogram).

Creating an ethogram begins with Step 1—reading the transcriptions created for each behavioral element in the taxonomy. Step 2 involves writing narrative text that describes in rich detail the behavior, the conditions and consequences of its occurrences, its range and variation, and its patterns. Particular attention will be directed toward incorporating the environmental and interactional contexts. This inductive descriptive analysis provides an important foundation for establishing what there is to explain and manage in real-life occurrences. Without it clinical researchers run the risk of focusing on insignificant behavioral elements, sequences, or missing or misinterpreting a phenomenon of significance altogether (Morse, 1990).

Credibility/Validity of Findings and Limitations

Internal validity or credibility of the findings from this analytic approach is strengthened in the present proposed research due to the following features: 1) Videotaping and field observations will be conducted by a psychiatric nurse social scientist investigator specifically trained in these methods. 2) The Research Assistant (RA) will receive additional training from the Principal Investigator (PI) to adapt his/her skill and knowledge to the elderly population in this research. The PI will accompany the RA into the study setting for early videotaping and will monitor videotaping thereafter. 3) Videotaping is the superior method for observing behavior. It provides the tunnel vision necessary to capture the nuances of a patient's posture, gait, gestures, and verbal patterns of communication—the aim of the present research. 4) Using videotapes that essentially stop time permits repeated checking of the data to ensure accurate interpretations. They may be staged in slow motion and/or are useful for frame-by-frame analysis. Such retrievable data enhances validity. 5) Data collection and analysis will go on concurrently as is expected in a design that aims to develop a taxonomy. Emerging analytic concepts will guide the sampling of additional data until saturation occurs to the degree possible within the constraints of this project. 6) Selected videotapes will be coded independently by both the PI and the consultant and discrepancies will be resolved if they emerge. The PI and consultant have years of social science experience both independent and collaborative landmark publications reflecting their expertise with this analytic method. 7) Data collection will occur at 78 points in time over a three-year period. This strategy aims to maximize the opportunities for observing behavioral variation over time. 8) Personal Notes (PNs) will be included in comments in the log. According to Schatzman and Strauss (1982) these notes encourage observers to consciously examine their own feelings, attitudes, and behavior. PNs along with research team dialogue will promote research reflexivity and minimize interviewer/observer bias. 9) External validity in this study design refers to analytic generalizability rather than the statistical generalizability in theory-testing study designs. As the taxonomy and ethogram become more comprehensive, their generalizability should increase for patients with AD. Quantitative research that aims to measure frequencies and to test the fit of the described behaviors with the levels of AD should follow. Limitations of the proposed research include the possibility that AD patients without prior diagnostic testing will not be included in the sample. A limitation of the data-collection strategy is that videotaped data depends on the researcher's judgment about who and what to videotape. We intend to address this by including a comparatively large number of hours of videotape and by documenting the full-range and variation of possible reactive effects of a videotaping schedule that will require reorientation of staff and patients to the data collector(s) and recording process every 2 weeks. In order to decrease staff and patients' possible discomfort from being videotaped some of the PIs donated time will be spent in getting to know staff and patients prior to and during the videotaping periods.

Title: Comparison of Prochlorperazine and Lorazepam Antiemetic Regimens in the Control of Postchemotherapy Symptoms

Authors: Sherri Simms, Verna Rhodes, Richard Madsen

Method

Sample: A convenience sample of adult oncology patients (n = 27; 15 women and 12 men) was recruited from a midwestern university teaching hospital and a veteran's administration hospital. To be included into the study, subjects had started their initial two cycles of chemotherapy (one of which was to be received as an outpatient) with one of four emetogenic agents. Subjects were excluded if any contraindications to the antiemetics were present. Ages ranged from 29 to 80 years (M = 56.96). The majority of the subjects were married (73.1%). Lung and breast cancers and lymphoma accounted for 85.2% of the cancer diagnoses. The majority (78%) of the 27 subjects received doxorubicin (Adriamycin) (M = dose $45.6/m^2$ cycle 1; $47.8/m^2$ cycle 2) and cyclophosphamide (Cytoxan) (M = $672.6/m^2$ cycle 1; $660.4/m^2$ cycle 2) with either 5-fluorouracil (5-FU) (M = $439.8m^2$ cycle 1; $381/m^2$ cycle 2) or vincristine (Oncovin) (M = $1.08/m^2$ cycle 1; $1.09/m^2$ cycle 2) as their chemotherapeutic protocol. (Where cyclophosphamide was the only study entry chemotherapy agent, n = 2, the M dose was $952/m^2$ cycle 1 and $955/m^2$ cycle 2.)

Instruments: PAST EXPERIENCE SCALE. Past experience, the subject's perception of past experience with another person treated with chemotherapy, was measured on the Past Experience Scale (PES) (Zook & Yasko, 1983). The PES is a single-item questionnaire with five response options ranging from 1 (extremely negative experience) to 5 (extremely positive experience). Patients are asked to rate their past experience with another person treated with chemotherapy on the 5-point visual scale. The past experience score was the number selected by the subject on PES.

INDEXING OF NAUSEA AND VOMITING. Total Nausea and Vomiting Experience was measured by the Rhodes Index of Nausea and Vomiting (INV) Form 2 (Rhodes, Watson, & Johnson, 1986). The INV Form 2 is an 8-item, 5-point, Likert-type, self-report tool. It measures patients' perceived nausea duration, frequency, and distress; vomiting amount, frequency, and distress; and frequency and distress from retching. Scores range from 0 to 4, 0 representing no symptom experience. Cronbach's alpha for the INV Form 2 was .98. Spearman's correlation coefficient (r = .87, n = 18, p < .001) was determined by comparing the ratings of patients with the rating of a family member the evening following chemotherapy. Scoring for the INV was the total of scores for nausea, vomiting, and retching for the 48-hour period posttreatment with the total possible score ranging from 0 to 32. ADAPTED SYMPTOM DISTRESS SCALE. Total symptom distress, a self-report of the occurrence and distress caused by 11 symptoms, was measured by the sum of the scores of 31 items on the Adapted Symptom Distress Scale (ASDS) Form 2 (Rhodes & Watson, 1987). The ASDS assesses the pretherapy and posttherapy symptoms of nausea, vomiting, pain, anorexia, sleep disturbances, fatigue, bowel elimination, difficulty in breathing, coughing, impaired concentration, lacrimation, changes in body temperature, alterations in body image, and restlessness. The 11 symptoms assessed by the ASDS Form 2 are further categorized into six symptom experience subscales; gastrointestinal problems (10 items), discomfort pain (7 items), respiratory problems (4 items), fatigue restlessness (6 items, concentration (2 items), and body image (2 items). The internal consistency reliability of the ASDS Form 2 is .91, as measured by Cronbach's alpha (Rhodes & Watson, 1987). A number value from 0 (no symptom experience) to 4 (most severe symptom experience) was assigned, with the total possible score ranging from 0 to 124. The ASDS Form 1 was adapted from McCorkle and Young's Symptom Distress Scale (1978); the ASDS Form 2 expanded Form 1 to better assess individual symptoms. Procedure: In this study, lorazepam was compared to prochlorperazine. Dexamethasone (Decadron), diphenydramine (Benadryl), and thiethylperazine (Torecan) were included in both antiemetic regimes as depicted in Table 1. Dexamethasone was given with both regimens to (a) deliver an enhanced antiemetic effect (Baker, Lokey, Price, Bowen, & Winokur, 1980); (b) decrease somnolence and thereby improve the patient's quality of life, because it permits the patient to function independently; and (c) promotes the maintenance of a normal appetite (Aapro et al., 1983). Diphenhydramine was given with both antiemetic regimens to prevent extrapyramidal reactions. Thietylperazine was included to standardize antiemetic treatment after discharge. All medications and dosages were prescribed by the physicians participating in the study, based on information from previous studies cited in the literature review and standard medical practice.

The study was designed as a double-blind crossover study. The staff pharmacist randomized subjects into one of the two antiemetic regimen groups; only he knew the regimen for a particular patient. Subjects gave written consent to participate in the study and were informed that they could withdraw from the study at any time or be withdrawn if any situation arose that potentially compromised their well-being.

Demographic information was gathered from review of the subjects' hospital records. Before the initial first cycle of chemotherapy, each subject completed the ASDS. After treatment, subjects completed the INV every 12 hours for 48 hours. The ASDS was completed again with the fourth INV, 48 hours after treatment. Subjects completed instruments on their own and returned them to the researcher in a self-addressed stamped envelope. During the second cycle of therapy, subjects received the antiemetic regimen not received during the first cycle and completed the tools as in the first cycle.

Source: Simms, S., Rhodes, V., & Madsen, R. (1993). Comparison of Prochlorperazine and Lorazepam Antiemetic Regimens in the Control of Postchemotherapy Symptoms. *Nursing Research*, 42(4), 234–239.

Discussion Guidelines

Discuss the following questions with your fellow students or colleagues.

1. Is the general design or approach of the study labeled (survey, case study, grounded theory, experimental, etc.), and is the reason for choosing the plan substantiated?
2. Are the exact steps necessary for data collection stated? Do the data analysis procedures address each aspect of data collection?
3. Is the research setting described if the setting is relevant?
4. Is the nature and size of the samples and the rationale behind these decisions clear?
5. Are the confounding variables addressed? Are any problems, errors in design, or limitations acknowledged?
6. In a quantitative study, are data-collection instruments discussed? Are the instruments consistent with the variable's operational definition, and is there empirical evidence attesting to their validity, reliability, and objectivity?
7. Is the method of analysis consistent with study questions and levels of measurement? Do the assumptions of the statistics fit the data that will be obtained?
8. In a qualitative study, are issues of scientific integrity such as credibility, confirmability, dependability, and transferability discussed?

Evaluation of a Timetable or Work Plan for Research Proposals

A work plan or **timetable** should clarify the overall flow of research-related activities. It should offer evidence that the nurse investigator has carefully and realistically considered the exact plans necessary to carry out the proposed study.

Directions

Refer to Figures 1 and 2 for examples of timetables for research proposals.

Discussion Guidelines

1. Does the timetable provide a clear, sequential statement of the operations that will be carried out?
2. Are the tasks or project activities included in the timetable?
3. Is there an estimate of the amount of time required and scheduled dates for each project activity?
4. Are personnel requirements for each activity listed?

Study Time Table

Activities	Months	Year 01	Year 02	Year 03
Phase I	16	1-6		
Employ Project Director	1	1-2		
Launch Interviews and Observations	7	3-9		
Type Transcripts	7	3-10		
Conduct Focus Groups	7	2-6		
Analyze Textual Data	8	4-13		
Interview and Observe	7	3-9		
Finalize Category Codes for Items	4	11-13		
Complete Analysis	3	13-16		
Phase II	18		13-30	
Finalize Q/L Items and Format	1		13-13	
Language Transparency Study	2		14-15	
Content Validity Study	2		16-17	

Figure 1. Timeframe. From Holzemer, W. and Wilson, H. S. Quality of Life Assessment in Advanced HIV Infection. 1994 Proposal.

Program Pen-Based Computers	2	17-18	
Validity & Reliability Study	6	18-23	
– Subset A Sensitivity	2	19-20	
– Subset B Test-Retest	2	21-22	
– Subset C Inter-Rater	2	23-24	
Data Entry, Coding, & Cleaning	6	23-28	
Data Analyses	3	27-29	
Complete Phase II	4	27-30	
Phase III	6		31-36
Item Development	1		31-31
Conduct Intervention	1		32-32
Assess the Take of Intervention	1		32-32
Collect Experimental Group Data	1		33-34
Data Entry, Coding, & Cleaning	2		34-35
Data Analyses	3		34-36
Complete Phase III	3		33-36

Timeline

TIMEFRAME   **FUNDING PERIOD**

                                 1987   1988

RESEARCH PROJECT	S	O	N	D		J	F	M	A	M	J	J	A
Month													
Data Collection	X	X	X	X		X	X	X	X	X			
Data Analysis	X	X	X	X		X	X	X	X	X			
Preliminary Report										X			
Report Revision											X		
Manuscript Submission to Research Journal													X
Final Report to FNF													X

Figure 2. Timeframe. From Hutchinson, S. Nurses who violate the Nurse Practice Act. Research supported by funds from the Florida Nurses Association, 1987.

47 Learning the Language Associated With Psychosocial Instruments

Many nursing studies rely on psychosocial instruments. To critique an article or to choose an instrument for research, nurses must be knowledgeable about these instruments, their assets, and limitations. First, however, the language surrounding their use must be understood.

Directions

Using the Glossary at the end of this book, match the definitions on the right to the correct terms on the left. Place the appropriate letter in the spaces provided. See how many you can identify before resorting to checking the answers.

Terms

_____ 1. **Objective measure**

_____ 2. **Psychosocial measures**

_____ 3. **Response set**

_____ 4. **Subjective measure**

_____ 5. **Semantic differential**

_____ 6. **Direct measure**

_____ 7. **Sorting techniques**

_____ 8. **Summative instrument**

_____ 9. **Projective tests**

_____ 10. **Proxy measure**

_____ 11. **Ranking techniques**

_____ 12. **Patient logs**

_____ 13. **Paired comparisons**

_____ 14. **Tests of knowledge**

_____ 15. **Ability tests**

_____ 16. **Rating scales**

Definitions

A. This tool easily and clearly measures variables such as age, height, and weight.

B. With this instrument, steps in a scale are selected and assigned numerical values (e.g., a Likert scale).

C. An example of this instrument is a written or oral test with items about the material covered in teaching.

D. Participants in studies using this instrument receive a stack of cards and sort them into piles based on a specified dimension (for example, preference, degree of stress).

E. This measure produces a count of something that stands for an object or quality.

F. These instruments measure psychological or social (not physical) phenomena.

G. A kind of rating scale where the ratings for each item are added to obtain the score.

H. An example of this instrument is asking patients questions directly or using a questionnaire about their perception of the adequacy of their knowledge about their diagnosis and treatment.

I. This instrument shows a tendency to respond to items in a consistent manner based on an irrelevant criterion, such as responding true to all items in a true-false test.

J. Participants rank certain objects on the basis of some property.

K. A type of rating scale typically used to measure attitudes. The concept to be rated is written at the top of the page, followed by a list of bipolar adjectives (love and hate, e.g.).

L. Participants record data systematically—open-ended or highly structured.

M. People choose between two objects or stimuli in each of a series of items.

N. Examples of these instruments include intelligence tests, achievement tests, and skill tests.

O. These tests request that the participant respond with awareness of certain facts or beliefs.

P. Participants are to respond to stimuli (often unconsciously), thus revealing aspects of their needs, conflicts, and personalities.

Answers to be found at back of book.

48 Reading Research That Uses Biophysiologic Variables

As a good consumer of research that uses **biophysiologic variables**, you should know how to critique such studies and you should have some specialized knowledge about them. The goal of this exercise is to have you ask questions that are specifically related to studies that use biophysiologic variables.

Directions

Read one or more of the articles listed in the references.

Discussion Guidelines

Discuss the following questions with a group of fellow students or colleagues.

1. Is the conceptualization of the phenomenon being studied the guiding force for instrument selection?
2. What are the independent and dependent variables in the study?
3. What are the biophysical data-collection instruments used by the researchers for each variable?
4. What issues threaten the validity of the measurements in the study?
5. What measures did the authors take to ensure reliability among the biophysical instrumentation?
6. Are the findings from the study sufficient to use as a basis for change in practice?

References

Bliss-Holtz, J. (1993). Determination of thermoregulatory state in full-term infants. *Nursing Research*, 42(4), 204–207.

Cole, F. (1993). Temporal variations in the effects of iced water on oral temperature. *Research in Nursing Health*, 16, 107–111.

Maloni, J., Chance, Zhang, C., Cohen, A. W., Betts, & Gange, S. (1993). Physical and psychosocial side effects of antepartum hospital bed rest. *Nursing Research*, 42(4), 197–203.

Meek, S. (1993). Effects of slow stroke back massage on relaxation in hospice clients. *Image: Journal of Nursing Scholarship*, 25(1), 17–21.

Simpson, T., Wahl, G., Detraglia, M., Speck, E., & Taylor, D. (1993). A pilot study of pain, analgesia use, and pulmonary function after colectomy with or without a preoperative bolus of epidural morphine. *Heart & Lung*, 22(4), 316–327.

Wilson, H. S. (1993). *Introducing Research in Nursing*, 2nd ed. Menlo Park, CA: Addison-Wesley.

Learning to Critique a Questionnaire

Developing a questionnaire is very complex, and many nurse researchers will never be involved in such an endeavor. However, all nurses can appreciate the process better by learning to critique existing questionnaires. Developing your critical nature will make you a better researcher and a better consumer of research.

Directions

Read the questionnaires "Home Support Needs of the Elderly Cancer Patient Receiving Outpatient Chemotherapy," "Demographic Information Sheet," "Chemotherapy Evaluation Scale," and "Chemotherapy Information Sheet."

Home Support Needs of the Elderly Cancer Patient Receiving Outpatient Chemotherapy

QUESTIONNAIRE

Sex: 1. Male
      2. Female

Age:_____

Race: 1. White (Caucasian)
       2. Black (Negro)
       3. Oriental
       4. Spanish American
       5. American Indian
       6. Other_____

Education: 1. 0-4 years
            2. 5-8 years
            3. High school not completed
            4. High school completed
            5. Post-high school, trade school
            6. 1-3 years college
            7. College completed

Are you: 1. Single
          2. Married
          3. Widowed
          4. Divorced
          5. Separated

Who lives with you?
1. No one
2. Husband or wife   Age_____
3. Children   Age_____
4. Grandchildren   Age_____
5. Parents   Age_____
6. Brothers or sisters Age_____

Continued on next page

QUESTIONNAIRE *(continued)*

7. Other relatives   Age_____
8. Friends   Age_____
9. Nonrelated paid helper_____
10. Others_____ (specify)

How many close friends do you have (people that you can talk to about your private matters or call on for help)?

1. None
2. 1-2
3. 3-5
4. 6-9
5. 10 or more

How many relatives do you feel close to?

1. None
2. 1-2
3. 3-5
4. 6-9
5. 10 or more

How often do you see a member of your family?

1. None
2. Daily
3. 2-3 times per week
4. Twice a month
5. Monthly

Do you see your relatives or friends

1. As often as you want to?
2. Are you somewhat unhappy about how little you see them?

Is there someone who would help you at all if you were sick (e.g., husband/wife, member of family, or friend) after chemotherapy?

1. Yes   Who_____
2. No one willing or able to help

If there is someone to help you if you are sick after chemotherapy, is the care adequate?

1. Yes
2. No

What side effects do you have within 1-3 days after your treatment? (circle all appropriate answers)

1. Nausea
2. Vomiting
3. Tiredness
4. Diarrhea
5. Sore mouth
6. Lack of appetite
7. Exhaustion

What side effects do you have 7-14 days after your treatment? (circle all appropriate answers)

1. Nausea
2. Vomiting
3. Tiredness
4. Diarrhea
5. Sore mouth
6. Lack of appetite
7. Exhaustion

Continued on next page

QUESTIONNAIRE (continued)

Is there someone who could take care of you
>   1. As long as needed?
>   2. Only for short time?
>   3. Now and then (e.g., fix lunch, take to doctor)?

If yes, who_____   Relationship_____

Is there someone to bring you to outpatient chemotherapy for your appointment?
>   1. Yes   Who?_____
>   2. No

If you are unable, is there someone to do (circle all appropriate answers)
>   1. Cooking?   4. Nursing care?
>   2. Shopping?   5. Dress you?
>   3. Housework?

Immediately after your treatment (1-3 days), are you able to (circle the answers that you can do)
>   1. Use telephone?
>   2. Get to places out of walking distance?
>   3. Go shopping for groceries?
>   4. Prepare own meals?
>   5. Do own housework?
>   6. Take own medicine?
>   7. Dress and undress self?
>   8. Take care of own appearance?
>   9. Walk with help?
>   10. Walk without help?
>   11. Get in and out of bed?
>   12. Take bath or shower?

If unable to do any of the above, who helps you?
>   Relationship_____
>   1. Lives with you
>   2. Lives outside your home

7-14 days after your treatment, are you able to (circle the answers that you can do)
>   1. Use telephone?
>   2. Get to places out of walking distance?
>   3. Go shopping for groceries?
>   4. Prepare own meals?
>   5. Do own housework?
>   6. Take own medicine?
>   7. Dress and undress self?

Continued on next page

QUESTIONNAIRE *(continued)*

8. Take care of own appearance?
9. Walk with help?
10. Walk without help?
11. Get in and out of bed?
12. Take bath or shower?

If unable to do any of the above, who helps you?

Relationship_____

1. Lives with you
2. Lives outside your home

Do you feel that you get enough understanding from your spouse or caregiver?

1. Yes   2. No

How many chemotherapy treatments have you had?_____

How do you get to outpatient department?_____

How often do you have treatment?_____

Do you receive help from any community agencies?

1. Yes   Name of agency_____
2. No

What additional help do you need that you presently don't have?

SOURCE: Marilee Wilkinson, RN, BSN, graduate student, University of Florida; Patient Care Coordinator, Hospice of Volusia.

Demographic Information Sheet

Please answer the following questions.

1. How long have you had cancer?
2. What type of treatment have you had in the past for cancer, and when?
3. Do you know the names of the drugs you will be receiving? If so, please name them.
4. In a crisis situation, who do you turn to for support? What is their relationship to you?
5. Do you know in what part of your body your cancer started? Please name.
6. If your cancer has spread to another place in your body, please name it.
7. Male_____ Female_____
8. What was your age in years at your last birthday?
9. What is your occupation?
10. What was the highest grade of school you completed?

Chemotherapy Evaluation Scale
"How I Feel About Chemotherapy"

Please indicate the number on each row that best describes your feelings about chemotherapy in relation to the words listed. Choose one number on each row.

For Example: If you were asked to describe your feelings about "SCHOOL" as either pleasant or unpleasant,

Where (1) is closely related to pleasant
(2) is slightly related to pleasant
(3) is equally related to pleasant and unpleasant
(4) is slightly related to unpleasant
(5) is closely related to unpleasant

pleasant   1   2   3   4   5   unpleasant

Choosing (2) would indicate that school was more pleasant than unpleasant, but not the most pleasant type of experience for you.

Looking at each pair of words listed below, please relate them to your feelings concerning "CHEMOTHERAPY."

Remember to choose one number for each pair of words.

GOOD	1	2	3	4	5	BAD
HOPEFUL	1	2	3	4	5	HOPELESS
HARMFUL	1	2	3	4	5	BENEFICIAL
WEAK	1	2	3	4	5	STRONG
COMPLETE	1	2	3	4	5	INCOMPLETE
SLOW	1	2	3	4	5	FAST
SUCCESSFUL	1	2	3	4	5	UNSUCCESSFUL
PASSIVE	1	2	3	4	5	ACTIVE
SAFE	1	2	3	4	5	DANGEROUS
COMFORTABLE	1	2	3	4	5	UNCOMFORTABLE

Chemotherapy Information Sheet

1. How do you feel about receiving chemotherapy?
Positive   Negative   Mixed
2. What have been your major sources of information concerning chemotherapy?
Nurses   Family   Friends   Newspaper   TV   Other
3. Has the information you have received about chemotherapy been helpful or harmful? Please describe how it has been helpful or harmful.
Helpful   Harmful   Neither   Both
4. Do you want to know more about chemotherapy?
Yes   No   Maybe

Continued on next page

Chemotherapy Information Sheet *(continued)*

5. What effects do you expect chemotherapy to have on your disease?
    Cure   Help Control Spread   Make Me Feel Better   None
    Other (please explain)
6. Are there things that worry you about taking chemotherapy? (Please name everything.)
7. What would *you* tell other people if they were beginning chemotherapy?
8. Do you have any additional comments (positive or negative) to make concerning your chemotherapy?

SOURCE: Fawbush, M. W.: *Attitudes Related to Cancer Chemotherapy: The Patient's Perspective.* Unpublished master's thesis, University of Florida.

Discussion Guidelines

Discuss the following questions based on a list originally developed in a classic book by Selltiz, Wrightsman, and Cook (1976), with a group of colleagues or fellow students.

A. Decisions about question content
    1. Is this question necessary? Just how will it be useful?
    2. Are several questions needed on the subject of this question?
    3. Do respondents have the information necessary to answer the question?
    4. Does the question need to be more concrete, specific, and closely related to the respondent's personal experience?
    5. Is the question content sufficiently general and free from spurious concreteness and specificity?
    6. Do the replies express only general attitudes and just seem to be specific?
    7. Is the question content biased or loaded in one direction, without accompanying questions to balance the emphasis?
    8. Will the respondents give the information that is asked for?

B. Decisions about question wording
    1. Can the question be misunderstood? Does it contain difficult or unclear phraseology?
    2. Does the question adequately express the alternatives with respect to the point?
    3. Is the question misleading because of unstated assumptions or unseen implications?
    4. Is the wording biased? Is it emotionally loaded or slanted toward a particular kind of answer?
    5. Is the question wording likely to be objectionable to the respondent in any way?
    6. Would a more personalized or less personalized wording of the question produce better results?
    7. Can the question be asked better in a more direct or a more indirect form?

C. Decisions about form of response to the question
    1. Can the question best be asked in a form calling for a check answer (or short answer of a word or two, or a number), free answer, or check answer with follow-up answer?

2. If a check answer is used, which is the best type for this question—dichotomous, multiple-choice ("cafeteria" question), or scale?
3. If a checklist is used, does it adequately cover all the significant alternatives without overlapping, and in a defensible order? Is it of reasonable length? Is the wording of items impartial and balanced?
4. Is the form of the response easy, definite, uniform, and adequate for the purpose?

D. Decisions about the place of the question in the sequence

1. Is the answer to the question likely to be influenced by the contents of preceding questions?
2. Is the question led up to in a natural way? Is it in correct psychological order?
3. Does the question come too early or too late from the point of view of arousing interest and receiving sufficient attention, avoiding resistance, and so on?

Reference

Selltiz, C., Wrightsman, L., Cook, S. (1976). *Research Methods in Social Relations*, 3rd ed. New York: Holt, Rinehart & Winston.

Reading Tables in Research Reports

50

Nurses are frequently put off by tables in research reports. Reading tables can help you as you skim articles and is necessary if you are reading at an analytic level. It is not a difficult skill to develop.

Directions

Read Tables 1-5, and answer the following questions.

1. Do you notice any trends?
2. What **measure of central tendency** did the author choose to use? Is it the "right" measure? If so, why, and if not, why not?
3. What is the **range** or **variability** of numbers in the table?
4. Are there any exceptions or "**outliers**" in the data? What does this suggest?
5. If possible, read the journal article references in the source line. Are the figures presented in the text consistent with those in the table?
6. Read the captions that accompany the tables. How do they compare with the results and discussion in the text?
7. Look up any unfamiliar statistics in a research statistics book. Were they used correctly in the tables?

Table 1 Patterns of siblings' participation in family's adjustment to hospitalization and selected characteristics of 59 families and hospitalizations

Characteristic	Active subgroups		Passive subgroups		
	Sib care (*n* = 8)	Self-care (*n* = 13)	High change (*n* = 12)	Moderate change (*n* = 14)	Low change (*n* = 12)
No. days in hospital (M)	4.0	3.9	3.0	4.2	4.5
Admission type					
% scheduled	50	31	42	43	33
% nonscheduled	50	69	58	57	67
No. sibling at home (M)	3.8	1.8	1.3	1.5	1.9
% with preschool children	75	0	45	71	67
% with one or more children >10 years	88	100	0	7	8

SOURCE: Knafl K: 1982; Parents' views of the response of siblings to pediatric hospitalization. Research in *Nursing and Health*, 5(1): 13-20.

Table 2 Parents' views of sibling responses to hospitalization of a child

Participation subgroup	Response			
	Negative	Concerned	No response noted	Total
Sibling care	1 (12%)	3 (38%)	4 (50%)	8
Self-care	2 (15%)	9 (69%)	2 (15%)	13
High change	8 (67%)	1 (8%)	3 (25%)	12
Moderate change	2 (14%)	3 (21%)	9 (69%)	14
Low change	0 (0%)	10 (83%)	2 (17%)	12
Total	13	26	20	59

SOURCE: Knafl K: 1982; Parents' views of the response of siblings to pediatric hospitalization. Research in *Nursing and Health,* 5(1): 13-20.

Table 3 Mean values for dependent measures by group over time

Dependent Measures	Preoperative Day		Operative Day		Postoperative Day 1		Postoperative Day 2	
	X	SD	X	SD	X	SD	X	SD
EMG in mcvs.								
Experimental	1.20	1.1	1.41	0.5	1.27	1.4	1.40	1.3
Control	1.35	1.2	1.94	1.0	1.54	1.0	1.12	0.4
Sensory rating								
Experimental	0.75	1.8	5.65	1.6	1.37	2.1	4.32	0.8
Control	0.76	1.9	5.40	3.39	4.24	1.6	5.50	2.4
Distress rating								
Experimental	0.58	1.4	2.95	2.4	1.00	22.0	4.40	0.4
Control	0.32	0.8	5.85	1.3	5.04	2.5	5.38	2.0
Potent Analgesic Use in mg of morphine								
Experimental			11.17	7.1	18.33	15.9	10.92	7.0
Control			33.58	29.7	46.03	34.7	24.33	23.8

SOURCE: Wells N: 1982; The effect of relaxation on postoperative muscle tension and pain. *Nursing Research,* 31(4): 236–238.

Table 4 Expectant parents' importance rankings of obstetrician characteristics: Before childbirth

Overall Rank[a]	Item[b]	Wife Rank (n = 22)	Husband Rank (n = 22)	Difference
1	Listen to and answer questions	2.0	1.0	1.0
2	Opportunity to ask questions	1.0	2.5	1.5
3	Inform about treatment risks	4.0	2.5	1.5
4	Favor father in delivery room	3.0	4.0	1.0
5	Favor minimum use of drugs	6.0	5.0	1.0
6	Favor prepared childbirth	5.0	7.0	2.0
7	Be a specialist, not a GP	8.0	6.0	2.0
8	Be friendly and talkative	7.0	10.0	3.0*
9	Give gentle examinations	10.5	9.0	1.5
10	Friendly office nursing staff	13.5	8.0	5.5*
11	Support breast feeding	9.0	11.0	2.0
12	Return calls quickly	10.5	12.5	2.0
13	Get appointment quickly	12.0	12.5	0.5
14	Reasonable fees	13.5	18.0	4.5*
15	More than 5 years experience	19.0	14.0	5.0*
16	Recommended by another doctor	16.0	16.0	0.0
17	Recommended by friend	20.0	15.0	5.0*
18	Trained at well-known school	15.0	22.0	7.0*
19	Encourage rooming-in	18.0	19.5	1.5
20	Encourage husband in office	17.0	21.0	4.0*
21	Office close to home	21.0	19.5	1.5
22	Short wait in office	23.0	17.0	6.0*
23	Payments on installment plan	22.0	23.0	1.0
24	Be male, not female	24.0	24.0	0.0

Note: all analyses performed on means computed from categorical rankings.

[a] Items ordered using overall mean ranks

[b] Each item preceded by the phrase "Of what importance was it in selecting a doctor that . . ."

*$p < .05$.

SOURCE: Brien M, Haverfield N, Shanteau J: 1983; How Lamaze-prepared expectant parents select obstetricians. *Res Nurs Health* 6:143–150.

Table 5 Number of patient responses, means, and standard deviations for samples of diabetic patients

	Number of patient responses		Scale means		Scale standard deviations	
	Phase I	Phase II	Phase I	Phase II	Phase I	Phase II
Control of effects of diabetes	156	92	3.44	3.42	.64	.65
Barriers to following diet	156	91	2.46	2.53	.72	.76
Social support for diet	156	91	3.37	3.48	.85	.95
Barriers to taking medication	113	79	1.80	1.61	.45	.59
Impact of job on therapy	83	49	2.04	1.98	.61	.62
Commitment to the benefits of therapy	155	91	3.91	3.81	.48	.58

SOURCE: Given, C et al: (1983). Development of scales to measure beliefs of diabetic patients. *Res Nurs Health*, 6(3), 127–141.

Discussion Guidelines

Discuss your answers to each question with fellow students or colleagues. Consult Wilson's *Introducing Research in Nursing* (1993) for help if you need it.

Reference

Wilson, H. S. (1993). *Introducing Research in Nursing*. 2e Menlo Park, CA: Addison-Wesley.

51 ## Comparison of Traditional Research With Field Research

Traditional **deductive research** and **field research** arise from different philosophic perspectives; they are different in their approach and in the phases of the research process.

Directions

Reread the introduction to this part and the definitions of deductive research and field research in the Glossary, then read the following statements and put the appropriate letter identifying the type of research (**A** for Traditional Deductive Research; **B** for Field Research) in the blank spaces provided.

_____ 1. Studies and/or generates many propositions

_____ 2. Is a linear process

_____ 3. Tests hypotheses

_____ 4. Generates hypotheses

_____ 5. Generates middle-range (substantive) theories

_____ 6. Generates concepts

_____ 7. Follows precise steps for data collection and analyses

_____ 8. Cyclical research process

_____ 9. Literature review or theoretical framework leads to research question or hypotheses

_____10. Data analysis begins immediately, occurs throughout the research process

_____11. Literature review is initially general, becomes more specific after the research findings are clearly outlined and described

Answers to be found at the back of the book.

Contrasting Qualitative with Quantitative Research

For a clearer understanding of **qualitative research**, it is helpful to contrast it to the quantitative approach. The differences in these two research methods are philosophical as well as methodological.

Directions

Pairs of terms are listed below. Each describes an aspect of either the qualitative or quantitative approach. Label the terms representing qualitative research with an **L** and the ones representing quantitative research with an **N**.

1. ____Soft science
   ____Hard science

2. ____Focus: concise and narrow
   ____Focus: complex and broad

3. ____Reductionistic
   ____Holistic

4. ____Subjective
   ____Objective

5. ____Reasoning: dialectic, inductive
   ____Reasoning: logistic, deductive

6. ____Basis of knowing: cause and effect relationships
   ____Basis of knowing: meaning, discovery

7. ____Theory: tested
   ____Theory: developed

8. ____Shared interpretation
   ____Control

9. ____Communication and observation
   ____Instruments

10. ____Basic element of analysis: numbers
    ____Basic element of analysis: words

11. ____Individual interpretation
    ____Statistical analysis

12. ____Emphasis on uniqueness
    ____Emphasis on generalization

13. ____Consider data first, then develop multiple hypotheses.
    ____Start with hypotheses derived from existing literature.

14. ____Study many propositions. Proceed through a multidimensional, "molecular" process.
    ____Study a few propositions. Proceed through a linear process.

15. ____Gather and analyze data simultaneously.
    ____Proceed through linear steps for data collection and analysis.

16. ____Test, confirm, or refute hypotheses.
    ____Generate concepts, propositions, and middle range theories.

References

Burns, N., & Grove, S. (1993). *The practice of nursing research. Conduct critique and utilization.* Philadelphia: W.B. Saunders.

Wilson, H. S. (1993). *Introducing Research in Nursing* (2nd ed.) Redwood City, CA: Addison-Wesley Nursing.

Adapted from: Joanne Weiss, MNS, ARNP
                  Doctoral Student
                  College of Nursing
                  University of Florida

The Language of Field Research

The language used in **field research** is considerably different from that used in traditional **hypothesis-testing research**. This exercise will make the new words meaningful. Use the Glossary as often as is necessary.

Directions

Match the definitions in the column on the right with the appropriate terms on the left. Place the appropriate letter in the spaces provided on the left.

Terms

_____ 1. The **field**

_____ 2. **Gatekeeper**

_____ 3. **Access**

_____ 4. **Entrée**

_____ 5. **Unstructured interview**

_____ 6. **Focused interview**

_____ 7. **Participant observation**

_____ 8. **Reciprocity**

_____ 9. **Informants/participants/** actors

_____ 10. **Diary** or log

_____ 11. "Casting a wide net" (Douglas, 1976, p. 195)

_____ 12. **Document analysis**

Definitions

A. A method of data collection and a role that, depending on the choice of the researcher, ranges on a continuum from complete participant to complete observer.

B. Getting to the peoples' hearts . . . getting them to open up and share their thoughts and feelings with the researcher.

C. An informant's written account of his or her experience.

D. The social-psychological areas where the investigator gathers data to find answers in the central area of inquiry.

E. Types of positioning by field researchers while observing. They include staying put, moving around the setting to observe in different locations, and following someone during the course of a day or an experience.

F. The sharing and exchange that occurs implicitly or explicitly between researcher and informants (participants).

G. This type of interview requires an outline of topics that the investigator intends to cover with each subject. However, the interviewer and subject may deviate

_____13. **Single, multiple**, and **mobile** positioning

_____14. **Field notes**

_____15. **Theoretical notes**

_____16. **Personal notes**

_____17. **Methodological notes**

_____18. **Introspection**

_____19. **Case study**

_____20. **Case history**

_____21. **Triangulation**

_____22. **Process consenting**

_____23. **Narratives**

_____24. **Bracketing**

_____25. **Reflexive**

Answers to be found at the back of the book.

from the prepared agenda to relevant thoughts as the conversation unfolds.

H. People who "control" access to social situations such as the head nurse of the labor and delivery suite and the secretary of medical records.

I. People who are in the social situations studied. In traditional research they are called subjects.

J. Talking to all kinds of people and investigating all kinds of settings associated with the phenomenon in question.

K. Interviews that stress the interviewee's definition of the situation and that let the interviewee introduce the notions of what he or she considers to be relevant instead of relying on the investigator's notions of relevance.

L. The ability of the field researcher to look within himself or herself and be reflective and analytical.

M. The goal here is to get the fullest possible story for its own sake. Findings are interpreted within theory, thus demonstrating how theory can be used to understand human experience.

N. Instructions to oneself, critiques of one's tactics, and reminders about methodological approaches that might be fruitful.

O. An in-depth investigation of a patient, a community group, or an institution like a hospital or clinic. The focus is on description, verification, or development of theory.

P. "A continuous process of establishing and developing relationships not only with a chief host, but with a variety of on-site persons" (Schatzman & Strauss, 1982, p. 22).

Q. The part of field notes that are purposeful attempts to derive meaning from observations. The researcher infers, conjectures, and hypothesizes in order to build an analytic science.

R. The analysis of documents that are relevant to the research study such as informants' diaries, hospital staffing patterns, video tapes, and nurses' notes.

S. Notes about one's own reactions, reflections, and experiences.

T. Written on transcribed observations and interviews usually kept in a certain form such as typed double spaced with a wide left-hand margin for data analysis and a heading including date, time, and place.

U. Refers to stories people tell about their experiences.

V. The type of consent used in qualitative research whereby the researcher obtains consent throughout the research process.

W. The introspective process used by the researcher throughout the study. The aim is to decrease bias and to gain insight about the researcher's involvement in the unfolding research process.

X. In qualitative research this refers to data from several sources, e.g., interviews, documents, and participant observation. It also may refer to the use of several researchers, several theories, and/or several methods. These strategies aim to enhance credibility, transferability and dependability.

Y. This term is most often used with phenomenology; it refers to setting aside the researcher's beliefs and perceptions about the area under study in an aim to diminish researcher bias.

Learning the Language of Qualitative Analysis

This exercise will acquaint you with the new language of qualitative analysis. Use the Glossary as a resource.

Directions

Match the correct letter of the definitions on the right with the correct terms on the left. Place the appropriate letters in the spaces provided.

Terms

_____ 1. **Analysis**

_____ 2. **Qualitative analysis**

_____ 3. **Content analysis**

_____ 4. **Descriptive statistics**

_____ 5. **Symbolic interactionism**

_____ 6. **Substantive theory**

_____ 7. **Formal theory**

_____ 8. **Cognitive maps**

_____ 9. **Straight description**

_____10. **Analytic description**

_____11. **Grounded theory**

_____12. **Intersubjectivity**

_____13. **"Lived experience"**

_____14. **Exemplars**

_____15. **Paradigm cases**

_____16. **Constitutive patterns**

_____17. **Dense**

_____18. **Basic social psychological process**

_____19. **Basic social psychological problem**

Definitions

A. This uses important categories from existing literature to organize data.

B. Rather than looking for objective fact, researchers examine their own perspective and interactions as both a source of data and as an analytic strategy.

C. This is the philosophy of science on which qualitative research is based. The implications are that research should be conducted in a natural setting; reality and truth depend on the way people define them; the research process itself is a source of data and analytic ideas.

D. These are visual models or diagrams of categories and relationships in the analysis.

E. This is the non-numerical organization and interpretation of data in order to discover patterns, themes, forms, and qualities found in field notes, interview transcripts, open-ended questionnaires, journals, diaries, documents, and case studies.

F. A theory grounded in empirical data. The researcher uses a method of constant comparison and coding to develop a complex explanation of conditions, consequences, strategies, phases, stages, ranges, and other relationships among the classes of variables discovered in the data.

G. A grand theory that explains how something occurs under a great variety of circumstances.

H. This involves devising novel categories suggested to the analyst by "interrogating" the data to organize it.

I. A middle-range theory that explains something under a specific set of conditions.

J. Numbers that report the frequency and distribution of categories assigned to the data.

K. The separation of data into parts for the purpose of answering a research question and communicating that answer to others.

L. A specific procedure for analyzing unstructured qualitative data. It is one way of categorizing verbal or behavioral data, and it requires analytic thinking and creativity in the researcher.

M. A core variable(s) that accounts for most of the variation in interaction in a grounded theory study.

N. A criterion for evaluation in grounded theory and other qualitative studies. The terms refers to the goal of richness and complexity that involves numerous concepts, properties, dimensions, phases etc.

O. Used in Heideggerian hermeneutics, these refer to participant stories that may be used in their entirety because they are especially vivid and reveal particular patterns of meaning.

P. In grounded theory studies the often unarticulated problem that a group faces in their daily lives/work. This problem is resolved by a basic social psychological process.

Q. Used in phenomenology and hermeneutics this term refers to the study of selected experience as it is lived by individuals. Such experiences are often obscured or "veiled."

R. Used in Heideggerian hermeneutics these refer to short stories or vignettes that capture meanings in situations or contexts.

S. Used in Heideggerian hermeneutics these refer to patterns that transcend and link the themes in a given study.

Answers to be found at back of book.

55 Distinguishing Among Types of Qualitative Research

There are many different types of qualitative research—**grounded theory, ethnography, phenomenology, ethnoscience, hermeneutics, historical inquiry**, and **ethical inquiry**, to name a few. The following statements describe the different methods.

Understanding the differences among qualitative methods is necessary to adequately critique qualitative research and to conduct a qualitative study.

Directions

Match the letter of the correct statement to the appropriate method at left. Place your answers in the space provided.

_____ 1. **Grounded Theory**

_____ 2. **Ethnography**

_____ 3. **Phenomenology**

_____ 4. **Ethnoscience**

_____ 5. **Hermeneutics**

_____ 6. **Historical Inquiry**

_____ 7. **Ethical Inquiry**

_____ 8. **Feminist Inquiry**

_____ 9. **Critical Social Theory**

_____ 10. **Case Study**

A. This method has its intellectual roots in anthropology and aims to describe particular cultures or subcultures, e.g., the critical-care unit, a psychiatric hospital, a barrio in Miami.

B. This method has its intellectual roots in philosophy and focuses on in-depth descriptions of the lived experience of selected people, e.g., women who are survivors of incest, children who have been diagnosed with cancer.

C. This method relies on documents, records, film, and, if possible, oral reports from involved people. The research question aims to gather data to interpret a past event based on a variety of evidence.

D. This method has its intellectual roots in the philosophy of Martin Heidegger and also focuses on lived experience. However, rather than presenting in-depth descriptions, the research report relies on paradigm cases, exemplars, and constitutive patterns.

E. This method aims to understand dilemmas in clinical practice, e.g., whether to resuscitate a patient or not, by using selected principles and theories and applying them to a particular case.

F. This method, derived from sociology, aims to generate a substantive theory, a theory about an empirical area of inquiry, e.g., women who repetitively contract sexually transmitted diseases, people who have had "out of body" experiences. The theory is integrated around a core variable.

G. This method derives from anthropology and is concerned with cultural knowledge. The aim is to understand the meaning of things as understood by participants; the meanings are explicated in categories or taxonomies.

H. This is an approach more than a specific method. Its aim is to understand the studied phenomena, to question the status quo, to search for alternatives that foster autonomy and responsibility. This approach emphasizes critical analysis of nursing, research, and practice.

I. This is an approach more than a method. It values studying a problem relevant to women, engaging with the female participants, and focusing on their experiences in context.

J. This provides an in-depth analysis of an individual, a family, a social setting or group conducted under natural conditions.

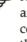

56 Ascertaining the Purposes of Qualitative Analysis in Nursing Research

According to experts, **qualitative analysis** has four purposes: exploration and description, accounting for and illustrating quantitative findings, discovery and explanation, and extension of **theory**. For assistance in doing this exercise, see Wilson, 1993, Table 11-2, p. 229.

Directions

Read selections from the materials referenced in this exercise.

Discussion Guidelines

Use the following questions as a guide to discuss each article with a group of fellow students or colleagues.

1. What is the purpose of the article? Is this clearly identified?
2. What are the research questions? Are they clearly identified?
3. What are the methods used? Could they be replicated?
4. What are the outcomes of the study?
5. Do the research questions, methods, and outcomes fit together logically with each other?

References

Aroian, J. A. (1990). A model of psychological adaptation to migration and resettlement. *Nursing Research, 39*(1), 5–10.

Brown, M. A., & Powell-Cope, G. (1993). Themes of loss and dying in caring for a family member with AIDS. *Research in Nursing and Health, 16*(3), 179–191.

Hutchinson, S., & Wilson, H. S. (1985). Americans on safari: An illustration of cultural complexity. *Public Health Nursing, 2*, 5–10.

Kondura, L. L. (1993). A Heideggerian hermeneutical analysis of survivors of incest. *Image: Journal of Nursing Scholarship, 25*(1), 11–16.

Thorne, S. E., & Robinson, C. A. (1989). Guarded alliance: Health care relationships in chronic illness. *Image: Journal of Nursing Scholarship, 21*(3), 153–57.

Wilson, H. S. (1993). Qualitative analysis. In: *Introducing Research in Nursing,* 2nd ed. Redwood City, CA: Addison-Wesley.

57 ## Critiquing the Reliability and Validity of a Study Using Content Analysis

  Content analysis is a specific procedure for analyzing qualitative data. It is one way of categorizing verbal or behavioral data, and it requires analytic thinking and creativity in the researcher. It has been criticized for its susceptibility to problems of **validity** and **reliability**. This exercise will help you look critically at the reliability and validity of using content analysis.

Directions

Read the classic article, "The meaning of current dance forms to adolescent girls: An exploratory study," In H. Kelly (1968). *Nursing Research*, November/December 1968, Vol. 17, pp. 513–519.

Discussion Guidelines

Discuss the following questions with a group of fellow students or colleagues.

1. How personal and idiosyncratic are the categories?
2. Would another researcher independently come up with the same ones?
3. Are the categories really mutually exclusive?
4. How clear are the instructions for placing a response into a code?
5. How reliable is the coding?
6. What checks did the researcher include on the reliability and thoroughness of coding?
7. Do the categories at least have face validity?
8. What kind of evidence is presented to establish face validity?
9. Do the content analysis categories meet other necessary criteria such as homogeneity, inclusiveness, usefulness, and mutual exclusiveness?

Understanding Ethnography

Ethnography is a qualitative research method useful in helping the nurse researcher understand the patient's culture, from his/her viewpoint. The following exercise will increase your understanding of the ethnographic method. The references serve as a foundation for the exercise.

Directions

Match the definitions in the column on the right with the appropriate terms on the left. Place the appropriate letter in the spaces provided on the left.

Exercise

Terms

_____ 1. **Etic**

_____ 2. **Emic**

_____ 3. **Ethnography**

_____ 4. **Cultural domains**

_____ 5. **Taxonomy**

_____ 6. **Componential analysis**

_____ 7. **Participant observation**

_____ 8. **Inductive**

_____ 9. **Contrast questions**

_____ 10. **Structural questions**

_____ 11. **Thematic analysis**
(discovering cultural themes)

_____ 12. **Descriptive questions**

Definitions

A. The third type of ethnographic questions. These questions are designed to elicit differences that exist among the terms in each domain.

B. Making generalized conclusions from particular observations.

C. The work of describing a culture (a process); the description of a culture (a product).

D. From the people's view and experience.

E. Systematic search for attributes (components of meaning) associated with cultural categories.

F. An external generalized universal view.

G. A category of cultural meaning that includes other smaller categories.

H. A set of categories organized on the basis of a single semantic relationship.

I. Also called fieldwork; going to the social situation for the purpose of engaging and observing the people and the situation.

J. The first type of ethnographic questions. These questions aim to elicit a large amount of information in the participant's language. They encourage descriptive observations.

K. The second type of ethnographic questions. These questions are based on the semantic relationship of a domain with a cover term. They are asked over and over again, and are useful in making focused observations.

L. This analysis provides an overview of the cultural scene and conveys a sense of the whole.

Answers to be found at back of book.

References

Germaine, C. (1993). Ethnography: The method. In P. Munhall and C. Boyd, *Nursing research, A qualitative perspective* (pp. 237–268). New York: NLN Publications.

Spradley, J. P. (1979). *The ethnographic interview.* New York: Holt, Rinehart & Winston.

Spradley, J. P. (1980). *Participant observation.* New York: Holt, Rinehart & Winston.

Wolf, Z. R. (1993). Nursing rituals: Doing ethnography. In P. Munhall and C. Boyd, *Nursing Research, A qualitative perspective* (pp. 269–310). New York: NLN Publications.

Adapted from: Susan Leger-Krall, MSN, ARNP
                  Doctoral Student
                  College of Nursing
                  University of Florida

59 Critiquing Qualitative Research

Because **qualitative research** is relatively new to nursing, and because some people do research without adequate expertise in the methodology, some of the articles in nursing journals confuse, or misuse the methods. For qualitative research to be done correctly the philosophical foundations and methodological guidelines need to be integrated; the purpose of the research needs to fit the chosen method.

Directions

Read the reference articles and discuss the following questions with a group of colleagues or fellow students.

1. Does the author identify the particular qualitative method used?
2. Does the method fit the purpose of the research?
3. Is the language used to describe the purpose and the method appropriate and accurate?
4. Are the data collection strategies appropriate to the method?
5. Are the findings presented in a style appropriate for the research purpose?

References

Butler, N. (1986). The NICU culture versus the hospice culture: Can they mix? *Neonatal Network,* 35–42.

Criddle, L. (1993). Healing from surgery: A phenomenological study. *Image: Journal of Nursing Scholarship, 25*(3), 208–213.

Elder, R., Humphreys, W., & Laskowski, C. (1988). Sexism in gynecology textbooks: Gender stereotypes and paternalism, 1978–1983. *Health Care for Women International, 9,* 1–17.

Hays, J. (1989). Voices in the record. *Image: Journal of Nursing Scholarship, 21*(4), 200–204.

Hutchinson, S. (1990). Responsible subversion: A study of rule bending among nurses. *Scholarly Inquiry for Nursing Practice, 4*(1), 3–17.

Kayser-Jones, J., & Kapp, M. (1989). Advocacy for the mentally impaired elderly: A case study analysis. *American Journal of Law & Medicine, 14*(4), 353–376.

Kondora, L. (1993). A Heideggerian hermeneutical analysis of survivors of incest. *Image: Journal of Nursing Scholarship, 25*(1), 11–16.

Langner, S. (1993). Ways of managing the experience of caregiving to elderly relatives. *Western Journal of Nursing Research, 15*(5), 582–594.

Morse, J. (1991). The structure and function of gift-giving in the patient-nurse relationship. *Western Journal of Nursing Research, 13,* 597–615.

Smith, J. (1981). The idea of health: A philosophical inquiry. *Advances in Nursing Science, 3*(3), 43–49.

Evaluating the Credibility of a Grounded Theory

The goals and methods of discovering **grounded theory** are quite different from the goals and methods of **theory-verification research**. The criteria for critiquing a grounded theory and evaluating its credibility differ accordingly.

Directions

Read one or more of the referenced materials in this exercise that use grounded theory methodology.

Discussion Guidelines

Discuss the following questions suggested by Strauss and Corbin (1990) with a group of fellow students or colleagues.

Questions About the Research Process

1. How was the original **sample** selected?
2. What major **categories** emerged?
3. What were some of the events, incidents, actions, and so on (as **indicators**) that pointed to some of these major categories?
4. On the basis of what categories did theoretical sampling proceed? That is, how did theoretical formulations guide some of the data collection? After the **theoretical sampling** was done, how representative did these categories prove to be?
5. What were some of the **hypotheses** pertaining to conceptual relations (i.e., among categories), and on what grounds were they formulated and tested?
6. Were there instances when hypotheses did not hold up against what was actually seen? How were these discrepancies accounted for? How did they affect the hypotheses?
7. How and why was the **core category** selected? Was this selection sudden or gradual, difficult or easy? On what grounds were the final analytic decisions made?

Questions About the Empirical Grounding of the Study

1. Are **concepts** generated?
2. Are the concepts systematically related?
3. Are there many conceptual linkages and are the categories well developed? Do they have **conceptual density**?

4. Is much variation built into the theory?
5. Are the broader conditions that affect the phenomenon under study built into its explanation?
6. Has process been taken into account?
7. Do the theoretical findings seem significant and to what extent?

References

Hutchinson, S. (1990). Responsible subversion: A study of rule-bending among nurses. *Scholarly Inquiry for Nursing Practice: An International Journal, 4*(1), 3–17.

LeMone, P. (1993). Human sexuality in adults with insulin-dependent Diabetes Mellitus. *Image: Journal of Nursing Scholarship, 25*(2), 101–105.

Patterson, E., Douglas, Patterson, P., & Bradle, J. (1992). Symptoms of preterm labor and self-diagnostic confusion. *Nursing Research, 41*(6), 367–372.

Pickler, R. (1993). Premature infant-nurse caregiver interaction. *Western Journal of Nursing Research, 15*(5), 548–567.

Strauss, A., & Corbin, J. (1990). *Basics of qualitative research*. Newbury Park, CA: Sage Publications.

Wilson, H. (1989). Family caregivers: The experience of Alzheimer's Disease. *Applied Nursing Research, 2*(1), 40–45.

Constructive and Destructive Criticism

Often the idea of having one's work critiqued is threatening to nurse investigators. Critics can, however, attempt to ensure that a criticism will be constructive, thus encouraging the researcher to improve his or her work and to feel satisfied with the criticism received.

Directions

Read the following critiques and then proceed to the Discussion Guidelines.

Critique

Title: Decision Making in Caregivers for Alzheimer's Dementia Patients

Author: Nursing Study Section, National Center for Nursing Research

CRITIQUE: This is a qualitative study of the decision-making processes that occur in the course of caring for an elder with probable Alzheimer's Disease (AD). This is a very interesting and worthwhile study proposed by two investigators who are well-prepared to conduct this study, who have worked together before, and who have preliminary work supportive of the project.

To gain a sense of what the investigators mean by decision-making requires some effort. They talk around the term until well into the proposal, and it then becomes clearer that the focus of the study is primarily on the family caregivers' decision-making at all steps in the process of caregiving. However, there is never a clear discussion of what constitutes decision-making. It is also not clear that the study can achieve some of its specific aims, i.e., where it is clear that one can identify and describe relevant social-psychological, social-cultural, and contextual factors, it is not clear that one can explain them with regard to decision-making processes through the data that will be obtained. The study has the potential of describing what decision-making means to the patients, family caregivers, and health care providers involved, and the extent to which they identify and describe the other variables of interest as being related to the decision-making experience. There is no intent to question the appropriateness of the grounded theory approach selected by the investigators for their work, but when the purpose of the investigation is to generate hypotheses, an explanation must follow later.

The investigators review the AD experience from a number of perspectives that they plan to probe in their work. They also draw on related literature in caregiving outside the AD experience where it is relevant for the proposed work. At times, however, they merely mention the existence of an article without explanation as to what it offers to the background of their work. They use quotations without references. In addition, absent from the set of determinants of decision-making processes are several patient-related factors that are relevant to the diagnosis and management of AD patients; e.g., patient functional abilities (physical and instrumental activities of daily living); behavioral problems (wandering, aggressiveness, resistiveness); and availability of resources and services.

The preliminary work of these two primary investigators is a strength. Dr. Wilson has already interviewed 20 family caregivers and identified a number of processes that could be replicated in the proposed study. It is not entirely clear how the family caregiver component of the proposed study differs from, or has derived benefit from, the preliminary study. However, the fact that the pilot study was done and that meaningful results were obtained supports the probability of the successful execution of the proposed study. The proposal also broadens the study to include the perspectives of patients and professional caregivers as well. Dr. Hutchinson is also experienced in grounded theory research methodology, having successfully completed and published several studies. It would have been enlightening to know more about her work on decision-making in health professionals that seems most directly related to the proposed work. However, her study of teaming high school students with institutionalized elders also supports her preparation to conduct studies with elderly clients. The combined expertise of Drs. Wilson and Hutchinson is a strength of this work. The study aims are appropriate to the proposed qualitative methodology.

There is also a certain appeal in the bicoastal interinstitutional approach proposed by the investigators. Each happens to live in a state that has a disproportionate share of the older population. Thus, these two long-standing colleagues are reasonable collaborators on a project that grows out of their own interests and experiences. It is also appropriate that they use purposive sampling so that the array of characteristics shown on page 51 of the proposals are, in fact, represented by the subjects in their study. The concern is that they have omitted one potentially important contextual factor; i.e., geography. In the description of the proposed study sites, several of the other characteristics are confounded with geography and there would be no way to distinguish the importance of that variable. For example, the two day-care centers included in the study are both in Florida. The distinction of a religious institution is evidenced in only one site in Florida. There are also concerns about selection criteria in the sampling plan. The investigators have chosen to select persons as "probable" AD patients on the basis of Folstein's MMSE, by clinical examination, and by the "review of carefully abstracted patient records by a psychiatrist consultant who is…an…expert in psychiatric diagnosis." This does not really describe what the criteria for inclusion are. What level of performance on the MMSE is required? What kind(s) of clinical examination will be considered acceptable? And is the nationally known expert in psychiatric diagnosis (expertise that is documented in his credentials) also a nationally-known expert in the diagnosis of AD (for which there is no evidence in the credentials)? With the lack of clarity regarding this diagnosis to begin with, it would seem that an expert in AD might be a more suitable consultant than the person proposed.

There are also concerns regarding the selection criterion for the family caregiver, which specifies that the individual will have been in the role "full time" for a minimum of 6 consecutive weeks. The concern is the definition of "full time." Does the individual have to have given up their job? Does the daughter of the patient have to have left her family and moved in with the patient to qualify? Many of the issues of caregiving burden have surrounded that need of the caregiver to keep up with what was already a "full time" set of responsibilities and add the care of the AD elder to that. There is also some concern about how the requirement for the caregiver to be English-speaking will be defined in practice. Both geographic areas contain many immigrants and cultural communities that reinforce the use of the native language. This is a difficult problem since there are some problems of comprehension if persons with limited English-speaking ability are included, and problems of generalizability of the findings if they are excluded. Under any circumstance, there is a need for clarification. Finally, with regard to the sampling plan, it is not clear how a unique triad of patient/family caregiver/physician or nurse will be accomplished if the study site has only one (or perhaps none) such professionals and ten subject clusters are to be derived from the site. It would not be appropriate to interview the same nurse ten times. Nor would it be suitable to relate her one set of responses to the responses of ten patients and family caregivers.

While the proposal justifies the need for a qualitative theory generating naturalistic study of decision-making, the participant observation component is the most disappointing. This is especially problematic because the identification of contextual factors in decision-making (aim 4) is based on observations of context. One hour per informant simply is not enough to warrant conclusions based on direct observations. Furthermore, the context and comparability of observations are not outlined.

While it is acknowledged that the quantitative component of this study is really secondary, there are nonetheless criteria that would apply here. Namely, there is no psychometric information provided for the quantitative measures, and there is no indication that the sample size (n) of ten from each location has sufficient power to detect significant differences between sites. It would also be helpful if the investigators, on the basis of Wilson's preliminary work or from some other data base, could project the approximate proportion of patients from whom it is likely that direct data could be obtained. It is not clear, if these figures were in the range of 10-20 percent, that there would be adequate sampling to reach saturation, nor is it clear that combining the family caregiver's recall of what the patient might have thought or said is a sufficiently comparable data set to combine them. The analysis, particularly the integration of qualitative and quantitative data, lacks detail.

Critique

Title: The Use of Seclusion and Restraints in a City Psychiatric Hospital

Author: Anonymous

The two research objectives are not clear. The first is directly related to the literature review that has adequate up-to-date references on the type of study—seclusion and restraints in a psychiatric hospital. A problem exists in that seclusion and restraints are never clearly defined and both terms can have many meanings, i.e., wrist restraints, leg irons, or total body restraints. There is a big difference and the definitions need to be made clear.

The second objective is to ascertain if information about the use of seclusion and restraints will produce a significant modification of nursing practice. This objective is not related to the literature review; it seems to derive from the assumption that information (control charts) will have some positive effect on nurses' behavior (putting patients in restraints less often). Merely sending charts through the mail is not a strong experimental manipulation. The theoretical assumption for the second phase needs to be more clear. That is, why would head nurses be expected to have the care on their units altered just because control charts were sent to them.

The researcher has done a good job of integrating the current literature, providing an argument for the need for the study. Relevant variables are discussed. The present, rather scanty state of knowledge of the use of seclusion and restraints supports the researcher's choice of the descriptive survey phase of the study. Until there exists more consistent and in-depth knowledge about the use of seclusion and restraints, research should focus on gaining such knowledge through description. Hypothesis testing studies should come later.

The study's relevance is supported by the literature review. The use of seclusion and restraints is a vital issue in psychiatry today, since seclusion and restraints are major forms of control and/or Rx (depending on the philosophical perspective of the unit) and both evoke such strong emotional responses from patients and staff. For professionals concerned with the quality of patient care and the new legal focus on least restrictive care, this study will offer important information.

The problems with the method have been mentioned earlier. Reliability and validity are not at all clear and they should be. Reliability sounds like it is being confused with validity, but the information given is too vague for me to be sure. I do not know if issues of confidentiality or anonymity of participating hospitals are relevant, but if they are, they are not addressed. A final question concerns the use of variables that are inherent in the different levels of medical centers and that are discussed in the literature. Will any tests be done (correlations?) on system-related variables? It is not clear if or how such variables will be used. To use them in some way would strengthen the study. The Project Management Plan is logical and seems feasible. However, there is no mention of which control charts will be sent to the hospitals and when. Data for the Control Charts will be collected from the beginning of phase one. Which 3-month periods of charts will be sent in months 14, 16, 19, 22, and 25?

Discussion Guidelines

Discuss the following questions in a group of fellow students or colleagues.

1. How does the critic's language influence the critique itself? Find an example of a clear and concise sentence and an example of an ambiguous sentence.
2. Are the critic's points ever trivial?
3. Is there a hint of ridicule or phony flattery? If so, where?
4. Are the good points of the study emphasized?
5. When the study's weaknesses are identified, are there clear explanations as to why they are weaknesses?

6. Are practical suggestions for improvement offered to the researcher?
7. If you received either critique on your work, how would you feel? Motivated to continue your work? Ready to give up?

Reference

Wilson, H. (1993). *Introducing Research in Nursing.* (2e) Menlo Park, CA: Addison-Wesley.

62 A Group Experience in Critiquing Published Nursing Research

All nurses should be able to help investigators refine and improve their studies or proposals. Learning to critique with a group of fellow students or colleagues can be fun and useful in developing ideas.

Directions

Choose one of the studies suggested in the references that is of interest to your group. Read the study carefully alone, and take notes on how the study meets the criteria listed below. At a prearranged time, meet with your group for at least an hour and compare and contrast your critiques.

Discussion Guidelines

Use the following criteria (Wilson, 1993) in doing your personal evaluation of a nursing study and as a guide in your group discussion:

Criteria for Good Research
CLARITY AND RELEVANCE OF PURPOSE

1. Will the study solve a problem relevant to nursing?
2. Will the facts collected be useful to nursing?
3. Will the study contribute to nursing knowledge?

RESEARCHABILITY OF THE STUDY PROBLEM

1.* Can the problem be answered by measuring **empirical evidence** or **data**?
2.* Can the problem be stated as a question that involves the existence of a relation between two or more **variables**?
3. Is the statement of the problem clearly and specifically articulated early in the proposal or report?
4. Have the investigators placed the study problem within the context of existing knowledge and prior work on the topic?
5. Are the **hypotheses**, or research questions, explicitly stated?
6. Are the **concepts** or variables operationally defined so that the methods for measuring them could be replicated?
7. Are the limitations and assumptions of the study included and are they logically justifiable?
8. Does the problem statement accurately reflect the title of the study?
9. Are the study questions, or hypotheses, clear, specific, testable, and consistent with the study title, purpose, and subsequent literature review?

*Most fundamental criteria

ADEQUACY AND RELEVANCE OF THE LITERATURE REVIEW

1. Has the investigator selected references that logically pertain to the subject studied and the methods used?
2. Can the study design answer the study questions and control the **extraneous variables**?
3. Are the data-collection procedures reliable and valid?
4. Does the investigator demonstrate that the instrument is free from ambiguity, bias, or significant omissions?
5. Are the sources for and adaptations of nonoriginal data-collection tools provided?
6. If the data-collection tools are self-developed, are the processes for developing them and reports for establishing their **validity** and **reliability** included?
7. Are the techniques for data collection logical and practical ways of acquiring empirical evidence on study variables?
8. Does the researcher include checks to guard against possible errors in collecting, recording, and tabulating?
9. If the design was experimental, do you find evidence of control of extraneous variables, manipulation of **independent variables**, **randomization** in both sample selection and assignment of sample members to treatment groups, and replicability?
10. What attempts were made to keep research conditions the same for all sample members?
11. Did the investigator try to keep subjects and researchers who are recording outcomes ignorant of which intervention was being administered to whom?

SUITABILITY OF THE SAMPLING PROCEDURE AND THE NATURE OF THE SAMPLE

1. Did the investigator choose to use a **probability** or **nonprobability sample**? Why one or the other?
2. What strategies were incorporated to avoid collecting a biased sample about which no generalization could be made to the target population?
3. Is the sample representative of the **population** to which findings are to be generated?
4. Is the sample size large enough to meet the assumptions of any statistical test that may be used in data analysis?
5. Is the sample size large enough to reduce the **standard error**?
6. What are the descriptive characteristics of the sample, particularly with respect to any variables that might influence study findings such as age, education, sex, or physical or psychological condition?
7. What criteria were used to enter eligible sample members into a study?
8. How was **informed consent** obtained and the rights of the human research subjects protected? (For example, did each subject get a complete and honest explanation of the purpose of the research, what was going to happen to him or her in the process, and the use to which findings would be put?)
9. Were subject losses that were due to the result of lack of follow-up or dropping out detailed?

CORRECTNESS OF ANALYTIC PROCEDURES

1. Does the author specifically name the statistical tests supplied, along with the **probability** associated with significant values?
2. Does the author explain and provide references for analytic strategies for nonnumerical data?
3. Are the statistical tests used appropriate to the level of measurement (**nominal, ordinal, interval**, or **ratio**) represented by the data?
4. Is a distinction made between statistical and clinical significance?
5. Is the statistical procedure the right one to answer the specified research question?

CLARITY OF FINDINGS

1. Are interpretations of results clearly based on the data obtained?
2. Are reasons given for tabulating or presenting data in particular ways?
3. Can you detect error in any computations?
4. Are there any discrepancies between results presented in graphic form and results presented in the text of the report?
5. Do all the tables and graphs have titles?
6. Are the relationships of the variables in tables clear and easy to figure out?
7. Has the researcher distinguished between actual findings, on the one hand, and interpretations made by the researcher, on the other?
8. Are the findings explicit enough for you the critic to decide if the interpretations are justified? (For example, some authorities agree that conclusions of any kind cannot be drawn from return of less than 51% of the sample.)
9. Are minor or secondary findings overemphasized in the report and major or primary findings underplayed?
10. Are the findings clearly and logically organized?
11. Is the presentation of findings impartial and unbiased?
12. Do generalizations or conclusions go beyond the data collected or the population represented by the sample?
13. Are the recommendations for further research offered?
14. Does the researcher include unsuccessful efforts and negative outcomes?
15. Are limitations that might have influenced the results noted?

References

Dilorio, C., Faherty, B., & Mantuffel, B. (1992). Self-efficacy and social support in self-management of epilepsy. *Western Journal of Nursing Research, 14*(3), 292–307.

Hurley, A. C., Volicer, B. J., Hanrahan, S. H., & Volicer, L. (1992). Assessment of discomfort in advanced Alzheimer patients. *Western Journal of Nursing Research, 15*(5), 369–377.

McSweeny, J. C. (1993). Making behavior changes after a myocardial infarction. *Western Journal of Nursing Research, 15*(4), 441–455.

Muller, M. E. (1993). Development of the prenatal attachment inventory. *Western Journal of Nursing Research, 15*(2), 199–215.

Smyth, K. A., & Yarandi, H. N. (1992). A path model of type a and b responses to coping and stress in employed black women. *Western Journal of Nursing Research, 41*(5), 260–265.

Wilson, H. S. (1993). *Introducing Research in Nursing,* 2nd ed. Menlo Park, CA: Addison-Wesley.

PART 4

Conducting Nursing Research

✤ Preparing a Research Proposal

Contemporary nursing research often must rely on funding if it is to be conducted. Obtaining this funding and institutional approval to conduct research studies in nursing often depend on how well an investigator conveys the soundness and coherence of the logic of a study plan through a written research proposal.

A well-written research proposal relates a project to a scientific tradition or prior work on a question, describes and justifies study procedures, and presents the importance of possible findings and conclusions to the solution of practical problems or nursing's goals of building a scientific knowledge base. Because the exact format of guidelines for preparing a research proposal usually vary with the funding agency or review committee to which it is being submitted, the investigator should obtain an application packet or set of guidelines from the agency, institution, or committee before submitting a research proposal. The requirements of a study proposal are as follows:

1. Identify the most important priorities for study in your situation.
2. Become familiar with sources of private and public funding (and even intrainstitutional funding).
3. Match your proposed project with the missions or goals of funding agencies.
4. Work closely with representatives from a funding agency as well as with people in your own institution (**The Human Subjects Committee [IRB]**), who may become involved with any research project that is initiated.
5. Follow the guidelines as closely as possible for format, administrative approvals, number of copies, and deadline dates for proposal submission.

Guidelines for Research Proposal Writing

A single set of rules cannot apply to the variety of research proposal formats. However, following a few general guidelines for presenting your research will increase the likelihood that your proposal will be acceptable to those who read it.

1. Consider your audience, and write for strangers. Readers and reviewers of your proposal will not be as well-informed about your research area as you are. Be sure to explain everything clearly and logically and avoid jargon and abbreviations that might be common parlance in your specialty, but unfamiliar to outside readers.

2. Package your proposal so it is attractive. An attractive proposal conveys the message that you, its author, have taken the time to demonstrate its value. This care is communicated by paying attention to technical details such as proofreading for typographical, spelling, and grammar errors; by following the instructions for proposal submission; and by carefully matching your study with the agency's or organization's interests and commitments.
3. Balance detail and flexibility. A finely crafted proposal reflects a balance between sufficient detail, which will convince reviewers that a study is worthwhile and the nurse researcher has the ability to conduct it, and sufficient flexibility, which will allow the incorporation of any suggestions for improvement.

✤ Relating Your Study to a Theoretical Context

Whether we are consciously aware of it or not, **theories** affect our understanding of the events and behavior we encounter every day. In different situations we hear about systems theory, organizational theory, economic theory, learning theory, small group theory, psychoanalytic theory, and the like. Confirming, refuting, transcending, generating, and adding to theory is one of the major reasons for conducting research studies. Thus, researchers usually try to place their studies within an existing, related theoretical context of what has gone before. When you begin to read about theory in nursing, you will probably encounter a relatively new vocabulary, including terms like **concept**, **construct**, **proposition**, **model**, and so on. Use the Glossary and the associated exercises in this book to familiarize yourself with the vocabulary of theory.

Developing theories that can be confirmed in empirical research is a complex, laborious, and time-consuming process comparatively new to nursing. Since approximately the early 1950s, nurse theorists have been attempting to articulate concepts and propositions that are useful for research and practice in nursing. Nurse researchers must be prepared to comprehend and evaluate theories borrowed and adapted from other related disciplines, as well as to interpret and evaluate the evolving contributions to nursing's own theoretical base.

✤ Collecting Data With Psychosocial Instruments

As concepts and constructs become more solidly established in nursing theories and theories of human response related to nursing, an increasing number of nursing research studies employ psychosocial instruments, or tools, like **rating scales**, **semantic differentials**, **sorting**, **projective tests**, and **questionnaires** to measure **variables** or **concepts**. Since the process of developing and testing a research instrument is extensive and time-consuming, it is important to be aware of how to locate existing instruments and evaluate them for their relevance to a nursing study's goals, **reliability**, and **validity**.

Sources of Existing Psychosocial Instruments

If you have decided that your research study requires collecting data on some psychosocial **variable** or **concept** such as coping style, sense of well-being, health beliefs, family functioning, social support, or life stress, you can save yourself unnecessary effort by searching thoroughly through sources of existing instruments rather than attempting to create one yourself, especially if your resources or skills do not permit you to test adequately for reliability and validity. Once you know what variable you intend to measure, consult the following resources to locate an existing instrument:

1. Compendia (collections that describe and often provide a sample of an instrument) that feature specialized instruments (e.g., instruments specifically intended for use among the elderly).
2. The most current edition of *Tests in Print*, which includes a wide variety of published instruments.
3. Compendia of unpublished instruments.
4. Abstracts of recent works using instruments that have not yet been included in a compendium. Two classic sources of particular relevance to nursing researchers are *Instruments for Measuring Nursing Practice and Other Health Care Variables* (Ward et al., 1979) and *Instruments for Use in Nursing Education Research* (Ward and Fetler, 1979).

Evaluating Psychosocial Instruments

The criteria for evaluating any psychosocial instrument include at least minimal levels of reliability and validity. **Reliability of measurement** refers to the consistency, accuracy, and precision of the measures taken. Reliability is your assurance that you will obtain the same reading each time a measure is taken unless, of course, a real change in value has occurred. **Validity** refers to the relevance of an instrument; for example, does the instrument really measure what it claims to measure? Most texts on measurement theory go into great detail on the various types of validity and the methods that are used to establish that a particular instrument has it.

Judging the worth of a possible data-collection tool also involves other considerations that are best determined by conducting a pilot test. **Pilot testing** can establish the following:

1. How long it takes to complete the instrument or battery of instruments, thus shedding light on questions of feasibility and acceptability to study subjects.
2. Whether some items or questions are unclear or irrelevant, suggesting how congruent the instrument appears with the theoretical constructs or variables you are using it to measure.
3. Whether subjects find the instrument objectionable, upsetting, or inappropriate, giving you further knowledge about how easy actual testing will be to administer and whether you can expect a good return rate from study subjects.

Scoring Psychosocial Instruments

Scoring **psychosocial instruments** can be complex and full of errors unless you take special care to reduce the likelihood of their occurrence. If you intend to score instruments by hand, experts suggest that you develop what are called **templates**. These are cardboard or plastic overlays with holes in them that allow only certain items or scales to be visible. Scores for various scales or subscales are thus figured out separately.

Computer scoring reduces the time involved in scoring instruments and also the chance of making errors. Computers can check for errors in hand-scored data sets, and software programs exist that actually score tests, compile subscales from items, and calculate any one of a number of other transformations or presentations of the scores.

Patterns of unanticipated responses in data are customarily handled by establishing something called **decision rules**, which ensure that other unusual responses will all be scored in the same way.

Developing Your Own Test or Questionnaire

This Guidebook follows the well-accepted idea that the creative talents, insight, and energy of most beginning nurse researchers can be devoted more profitably to other steps of the research process than to the complex process of developing and testing new psychosocial instruments. If, however, you are unable to locate an appropriate existing tool, you should consult standard test books on measurement theory and instrument development and/or the guidance of an expert to create a plan for developing your own psychosocial instrument.

✤ Collecting Data on Biophysiologic Variables

Nursing research need not be concerned with variables that are exclusively psychosocial in nature. Many practice questions focus on variables like oxygen consumption, intracranial pressure, dyspnea, pain, urinary output, and wound healing. In such studies, where biophysiologic phenomena and variables are of interest, a wide range of instrumentation can be used. In some studies equipment is used to create the study's **independent variable**, such as equipment for oxygen administration, suctioning, or administering tube feedings. In other cases the instruments and equipment may be used to measure the **dependent variable**. Familiar examples include thermometers, scales, electroencephalogram tracings, Holter monitors, and strain gauges.

Selecting Instruments to Measure Biophysiologic Variables

The guiding principle for selecting instruments to create a nursing study's independent variable or measure the dependent variable depends on the conceptualization and **operational definition** of the phenomena being studied.

✤ Using Statistics to Analyze Quantitative Data

Statistics are valuable tools for analyzing numerical data to answer certain research questions. Understanding what statistical concepts mean, matching statistical procedures to study purposes and design, and knowing something about the assumptions necessary for using certain statistical tests are all competencies you will need to judge the credibility of findings in nursing research or to conduct research yourself. Unless you know the meaning of the statistical results you read, you risk basing your practice decisions on poor information.

Key Points on the Subjects of Statistics

Exercises in this Part introduce you to the application of selected knowledge about statistical analysis. However, they are not a substitute for a more comprehensive nursing research textbook or a good introductory statistics text. The following is a summary of some key points about statistics that, in combination with the Glossary and exercise References, can provide you with a beginning orientation to this topic.

1. Statistics are analytic tools that let researchers determine if something is more or less likely to occur according to the laws of **probability**. In other words, they tell you if something is or is not due to chance.

2. Understanding statistics requires that you understand the process of scientific measurement in which numerical values are assigned to the attributes or qualities of phenomena called variables.

3. Levels of data measured include **nominal** (naming), **ordinal** (ordering), **interval** (all possible measurements are equidistant from one another and ordered from low to high), and **ratio** (an interval scale that also has an absolute, rather than arbitrary zero point).

4. Knowing the level of measurement you are working with helps you decide which statistical procedures are appropriate.

5. If you are conducting your own study, it is a good idea to get statistical consultation early in the planning stage so you can anticipate how you intend to analyze your data.

6. Statistical tests fall into two major categories: **descriptive statistics**, which are used to summarize the characteristics of a data set, and **inferential statistics**, which allow a researcher to make inferences about a whole population based on data collected from a selected sample.

7. Inferential statistics are based on the assumption that the investigator has taken a **random sample** from the **population** or has a sample size large enough to assume a **normal distribution** of the variable under investigation.

8. The logic behind inferential statistics is that chance produces variation among groups. The statistical test is designed to reject this assumption and conclude with a specified level of certainty that any differences are due to the independent variable or intervention introduced by the investigator.

9. The formulas and assumptions about level of data and the **critical values** for various statistics must all be looked up in a statistics book in order to be used (or understood) well.

10. Advanced statistics such as **multiple correlation regression**, **analysis of covariance**, **factor analysis**, and **discriminant analysis** can be used when a study is trying to untangle complex relationships among three or more variables.

✤ First-Hand Knowing Under Natural Conditions: The Field Research Approach

Fieldwork's Philosophy of Science

The type of research variously called **fieldwork**, field research, **ethnography**, and **qualitative research** grew out of intellectual traditions in anthropology and sociology. The fundamental philosophical premise that is the basis for this approach to science is that people define their experiences differently under different conditions. The best way to learn about these varying realities is to directly observe the situation or social world under investigation and try to discover its own order or particular logic.

Data-Collection Tools in Field Research

Fieldwork as a style of scientific inquiry immerses the researcher in the processes of day-to-day life of the subjects or groups being studied. Thus, **the field** can be any social-psychological or structural area where the investigator uses strategies such as **participant observation**, or **semi-focused interviewing**, and **document analysis** to find answers to the central area of inquiry.

Strategies for Data Collection in Field Research

Answers to certain research questions are best obtained from one data collection strategy than another. For example, participant observation might be preferable to interviewing if you wish to study interaction over time; interviewing might be better suited to learning about patients' highly personal perceptions or experiences. Two criteria guide the field researcher in selecting data-collection strategies: (1) Providing for the most complete and accurate data, and (2) Being as efficient and economical as possible. The major methods used by field researchers for collecting data are:

1. Participant observation
2. Interviewing informants
3. **Unobtrusive** or **nonreactive methods** such as analysis of documents, written case histories, artifacts (e.g., toys children take to the hospital or personal objects the elderly select when moving to a nursing home).
4. **Focus groups**

In many instances field researchers will use all four methods to cross-check what they are finding using different data-collection methods. Each of the data-collection strategies listed has advantages and disadvantages. Completing Exercises in Part 4 of this book will familiarize you with techniques, language, and steps associated with field research and will introduce you to some of the unique responses that field research can evoke in the nurse researcher.

Field Research's Contribution to Nursing

Many nursing leaders agree that the essence of nursing research is everyday nursing practice because the business of nurse researchers should be to examine, describe, explain, and predict that practice. Answering clinical questions can generate the knowledge necessary to improve patient care. Field research, whether conducted in prenatal classes, self-help meetings, shift reports, or intensive care units, is particularly well-suited to gaining insights into the real world of daily nursing practice and can easily be incorporated into the practicing nurse's role and perspective.

Despite what seems to be its compelling potential for contributing to knowledge about real-world clinical practice, field research could be dismissed as journalism, or too subjective as long as field researchers fail to systematically and precisely describe both their methods of data collection and data analysis. "Hanging out" and "having insight" don't qualify as sufficient methodological descriptions, enabling another researcher to replicate a study.

✤ The Craft of Qualitative Analysis

When a research study involves open-ended, nonstructured, informal, nonnumerical data (such as those collected when using the strategies of field research discussed in the preceding section), the researcher must derive some meaning out of this array of what may seem like heterogeneous data. Studies involving such data and addressing questions about people's experiences under natural conditions employ techniques for analyzing the data that are quite distinct from the descriptive and inferential statistical analysis procedures described earlier.

Preparing Qualitative Data for Analysis

The qualitative analyst must develop a system for keeping track of what may be thousands of pages of field notes and interview transcripts. The following steps offer guidelines for organizing and filing qualitative data so that you can retrieve it as needed.

Steps in Labeling, Indexing, and Filing Data

1. Transcribe all handwritten field notes, taped interviews, and documents on $8\frac{1}{2} \times 11$ inch paper, leaving wide margins on the right-hand side where you later write codes or concepts for which the anecdote is an **indicator**. Usually typed data are entered into a computer using a software program like *Windows* or *Ethnograph*.
2. Label each page with identifying information using code names or numbers to protect the confidentiality rights of subjects and settings.
3. Make at least three duplicate sets of your data disk and keep them in different places (safe deposit box at bank, home, and work).

4. Set up a filing system so that you can block move the chronological narrative of field notes, for example, into different arrangements.

Types of Files

1. Organizational files keep track of people, addresses, phone numbers, and dates. Some qualitative experts call these "mundane files" because they help you keep track of mundane details.
2. Analytic files consist of separate folders for as many codes or concepts that seem to be emerging in your analysis of the data and the examples in the data that illustrate them.
3. Methodological files contain your reflections on any methodological problems encountered and the strategies used.

This manual system for filing qualitative data and for analysis of it has undergone major transformations as field researchers have substituted computer software programs and diskettes for the cardboard boxes of file folders that used to fill their shelves.

How to Write a Research Problem

63

Writing the research problem is the first procedure in the research process. Certain steps can be followed that will help refine your area of interest into a researchable problem.

Directions

The steps used to refine your problem are listed in the left column. In the right column, *write your own example for each step.* After completing the final step, you will have defined a researchable problem.

Steps	**Example**
1. State the discrepancy (between what happens and what you want to happen). For example, why do chemotherapy patients get nauseated every time I (the chemotherapy nurse) enter the room?	1.
2. Consider all the plausible obstacles, constraints, or explanations (e.g., fear, prior experience of nausea, fatigue, pain, no knowledge of what to expect, anger, concern about dying, concern over body image changes).	2.
3. Narrow the focus by selecting a few specific high priority variables such as prior experience of nausea and fear.	3.
4. Rephrase the question in conceptual terms. For example, will teaching relaxation exercises and self-hypnosis to patients prior to chemotherapy result in decreased nausea when compared to a group without the nursing interventions?	4.

Discussion Guidelines

Discuss your research questions with fellow students or colleagues.

1. Can you identify the discrepancy?
2. Are your selected variables high priority?
3. Is your rephrased question a researchable problem?

Doing a Literature Review

Your literature review should include six major types of literature: (1) relevant nursing research, (2) theoretical literature, (3) general and specialty nursing literature, (4) methodological literature, (5) research literature from other disciplines, and (6) popular literature. Of course, you may not always find related articles, but you should attempt to do a thorough search, usually with the help of a librarian and a computer.

Directions

Choose one of your research questions from the three previous exercises and do a computerized search on the topic. Read the articles and then divide them into the appropriate categories that follow, listing them in bibliographical form.

Relevant nursing research   1.
                                                   2.
                                                   3.
Theoretical literature   1.
                                                   2.
                                                   3.
General and specialty nursing literature   1.
                                                   2.
                                                   3.
Methodological literature   1.
                                                   2.
                                                   3.
Research literature from other disciplines   1.
                                                   2.
                                                   3.
Popular literature   1.
                                                   2.
                                                   3.

Discussion Guidelines

1. Into what category did most of your articles fall?
2. What does the answer to question 1 tell you about the nature of the existing knowledge on the subject? For example, are most of the articles research-based?
3. What do the answers to questions 1 and 2 tell you about the level of research question you should ask?
4. Write your research question at the appropriate level, based on your review of the literature.

Developing a Summary Chart

Summary charts organize groups of prior studies about research areas such as wandering in Alzheimer's Dementia patients or feeding problems in neonates. This exercise will help you develop your own summary chart on a problem that interests you.

Directions

Collect, via computer search or by skimming through the last few years of nursing research journals, several articles that examine the **biophysiologic variables** that interest you. Make a summary chart and identify the following information.

1. Authors
2. Source of their report
3. Purpose(s) of the study
4. Research questions or hypotheses
5. Independent and dependent variables
6. Measures and equipment that were used to quantify the variables
7. Study samples
8. Specific procedures described for the data collection
9. Major findings and conclusions

Discussion Guidelines

Go over the chart with a group of interested fellow students or colleagues and discuss the following questions.

1. What is your evaluation of each study; that is, what are the assets or limitations?
2. Are the designs similar or different? Does one design seem better than the others?
3. What are the different data-collection techniques? What are the problems with each? The good points?
4. How do the findings of the studies compare?
5. If you were going to carry out a study dealing with a similar problem, how would you do it?

Use of Theory In Your Literature Review

It is necessary for you to understand the types of theory and their varying degrees of involvement with the real world in order to determine their relevance when you are reading for your literature review. This exercise provides some guidelines that will help you analyze your readings.

Directions

Read several of the references provided in this exercise.

Discussion Guidelines

After reading the articles, discuss the following questions with a group of colleagues or fellow students.

1. Is this article presenting a **grand theory**, a **middle theory**, or an example of **abstracted empiricism**?
2. Could this article be used to derive **hypotheses** for testing? Give an example.
3. Does the article offer any sensitizing **concepts**?
4. Are the concepts generally global and ambiguous or clearly defined?
5. Is the focus general, very specific, or in the middle of the two extremes?
6. Does the article have any relevance for nursing education or practice? If so, what relevance does it have?
7. Could the **theory** be represented by a **model**? What would it look like?
8. What, if any, is the relationship of the article to theory?

References

Hutchinson, S. (1992). Nurses who violate the Nurse Practice Act: Transformation of professional identity. *Image: Journal of Nursing Scholarship, 24*(2), 133–139.

Koziol-McLain, J., & Maeve, M. (1993). Nursing theory in perspective. *Nursing Outlook, 41*(2), 79–81.

Lindgren, C., Burke, M., Hainesworth, M., & Eakes, G. (1992). Chronic sorrow: A lifespan concept. *Scholarly Inquiry for Nursing Practice: An International Journal, 6*(1), 27–40.

Moody, L. (1989). Building a conceptual map to guide research. *Florida Nursing Review, 4*(1), 1–5.

Sandelowski, M. (1993). Theory unmasked: The uses and guises of theory in qualitative research. *Research in Nursing and Health, 16,* 213–218.

Writing Level 1 Research Questions

Many interesting, researchable questions can be identified and cultivated into completed research studies from your clinical area, the literature, or nursing theories. The purpose of this exercise is to help you identify a Level 1 question of interest for you. Level 1 questions are used in **exploratory** and **descriptive** research and begin with the stem, "What," followed by a topic. Little specific information about Level 1 questions is found in the existing literature.

Directions

Observe, read about, or think about familiar problems in which you are interested. Then write several Level 1 research questions for your chosen problem. For example, "What do insulin-dependent diabetic patients want to know about their disease?"

Level 1 Research Questions

Stem	Topic
1. What . . .	do insulin-dependent diabetic patients want to know about their disease?
2.	
3.	
4.	
5.	

Discussion Guidelines

Discuss the following questions with your colleagues or fellow students.

1. Does each question have a **variable**? What is it?
2. Does each question have a **population**? What is it?
3. Is the problem researchable (i.e., does not request a "yes" or "no" answer or value or opinions)?
4. Is it feasible (possible and practical) to research the question?
5. Will the knowledge gained contribute to nursing knowledge or practice? How?

68   ## Writing Level 2 Research Questions

Level 2 questions look for a relationship between two **variables** and begin with the stem, "What is the relationship?" The literature review will not specify the precise nature of the relationship between the variables, but it will give you enough information so that you can make a conceptual leap in assuming that the relationship might logically exist.

Directions

After reading in your field or after thinking about your clinical experience, write some Level 2 research questions. For example, "What is the relationship of patient education to patient compliance in a cardiac rehabilitation program?"

Level 2 Research Questions

Stem	**Topic**
1. What is the relationship . . .	of patient education to patient compliance in a cardiac rehabilitation program?
2.	
3.	
4.	
5.	

Discussion Guidelines

Discuss the following questions with a group of fellow students or colleagues.

1. Does each question have two **variables**? What are they?
2. Does each questions have a **population**? What is it?
3. Is the problem researchable (i.e., does not request a "yes" or "no" answer or value or opinions)?
4. Is it feasible (possible and practical) to research the question? What are the problems you foresee?
5. Will the knowledge gained contribute to nursing knowledge or practice? How?

Writing Level 3 Research Questions

Level 3 inquiry assumes a relationship, either causal or influential, between two **variables** and begins with the stem "Why?" Your literature review will reveal theory (or other findings) that predict the nature of the relationship.

Directions

After reading literature in your field, write some Level 3 research questions. For example, "Why do self-care behaviors increase the feelings of well-being in patients with chronic illness?"

Level 3 Research Questions

Stem	**Topic**
1. Why . . .	do self-care behaviors increase the feelings of well-being in patients with chronic illness?
2.	
3.	
4.	
5.	

Discussion Guidelines

Discuss the following questions with your colleagues or fellow students.

1. Does each question have two **variables**, one that is predicted to be causal and one that is the effect, or outcome, variable? What are they?
2. Does each question have a **population**? What is it?
3. Does each question predict a direction? What is it?
4. Is the problem researchable (i.e., does not request a "yes" or "no" answer or values or opinion)?
5. Is it feasible (possible and practical) to research the question? What are the problems you foresee?
6. Will the knowledge gained contribute to nursing knowledge or practice? How?

70 Writing a Statement of Purpose

The statement of purpose answers the question "Why do the study?" Brink and Wood (1984) suggest that the purpose be written as a statement for a Level 1 study, as a question for a Level 2 study, and as a **hypothesis** for a Level 3 study.

Directions

Read the following three examples and then rewrite your own examples (two each) from the previous exercises into a statement of purpose for a Level 1, 2, and 3 study.

Example Level 1

In a study that asks the question "What are the eating habits of bulimics?" the statement of purpose can be expressed as follows: The purpose of this research is to explore and describe the eating habits of bulimics.

Your statement of purpose: 1.

                                  2.

Example Level 2

In a study that asks the question "What is the relationship between smoking and prematurity in primiparous mothers?" the statement of purpose is: The purpose of the study is to answer the question "Is there a significant relationship between smoking and prematurity in primiparous mothers?"

Your statement of purpose: 1.

                                  2.

Example Level 3

In a study that asks the question "Why does the teaching of self-care strategies increase the feeling of well-being in chronically ill patients?" the statement of purpose is: The purpose of this study is to test the hypothesis that chronically ill patients who are taught self-care techniques will have higher scores on feelings of well-being than those who do not receive the teaching.

Your statement of purpose: 1.

                               2.

Discussion Guidelines

Discuss the following questions with a group of colleagues or fellow students.

1. Do you agree or disagree that writing a statement of purpose adds clarity to your proposal? Why?
2. Look through the latest issues of *Nursing Research* and *Western Journal of Nursing Research*, or any other research journal to see how authors write, or do not write, their purposes. Which methods seem best to you? Why?

Reference

Brink, P., Wood, M. (1984). *Basic Steps in Planning Nursing Research, From Question to Proposal*. Boston, Mass: Jones and Bartlett Pub.

Writing Hypotheses

Brink and Wood (1984) identified three components that are essential to a well-written **hypothesis**: (1) the **experimental group**, (2) the expected result, and (3) the **comparison group**.

Directions

Look at the following example of a hypothesis and write at least two hypotheses from your literature review that you are interested in testing. Example: There will be significant declines in all functional dimensions (social, economic, mental health, physical health, and activities of daily living, ADL) in the 5-year interval following immigration.

1.

2.

Discussion Guidelines

Discuss the following questions with a group of fellow students or colleagues.

1. Do your hypotheses have the three components necessary for a well-written hypothesis? If not, rewrite the hypotheses to include the three parts.
2. What is the experimental group?
3. What is the expected result?
4. What is the comparison group?

References

Ailinger, R., Dear, M., and Holley-Wilcox, P. (1993). Predictors of function among older Hispanic immigrants: A five-year follow-up. *Nursing Research, 42*(4), 240–244.

Brink, P., Wood, M. (1984). *Basic Steps in Planning Nursing Research, From Question to Proposal*. Boston, Mass: Jones and Bartlett.

Defining Your Variables Operationally

Once your **purpose/question/hypothesis** is written with your **variables** clearly delineated, you need to write **operational definitions** for them. (Remember that variables are any factors that vary and that an **independent variable** can stand alone, whereas a **dependent variable** depends on another variable.) Operationally defining your variables requires that you clearly specify them, and indicate how you are measuring them.

Directions

Read the following examples of operational definitions. Then choose variables from your purpose/question/hypotheses from previous exercises, and write operational definitions for them. For example, an operational definition of age is: "The age of the subject will be asked during the interview session and will be recorded in number of years and months." An operational definition of sleep pattern is: "Sleeping electroencephalograms will be recorded over one 8-hour period, and the pattern will be assessed according to the Bannon Sleep Pattern Instrument."

Operational definitions from your proposed study:

1.

2.

3.

4.

Discussion Guidelines

Discuss the following questions with your fellow students or colleagues.

1. Are your definitions clear?
2. How will each of your variables be measured?
3. Could some of your variables be measured using several different methods? Why did you choose the one you did?

Reference

Wilson, H. (1993). *Introducing Research in Nursing,* 2nd ed. Menlo Park, CA: Addison-Wesley.

73 The Sampling Process

Sampling is a vital part of the research process, and the strategies for choosing your sample will influence your results and your interpretation of them. You must choose a **sample**, a subset of the **population**, and you must be concerned with how you can get the most representative or informative sample possible. This exercise is designed to help you choose the best sampling strategy for your study.

Directions

Match the letter of the appropriate definition with the type of sampling at the left. Place the letters in the spaces provided.

Type of Sampling

_____ 1. **Probability sampling**

_____ 2. **Systematic sampling**

_____ 3. **Cluster sampling**

_____ 4. **Snowball sampling**

_____ 5. **Expert sampling**

_____ 6. **Quota sampling**

_____ 7. **Stratified random sampling**

_____ 8. **Purposive, or judgement, sampling**

_____ 9. **Nonprobability sampling**

_____ 10. **Simple random sampling**

_____ 11. **Accidental, or convenience, sampling**

_____ 12. **Theoretical sampling**

Definition

A. Each individual in the sampling frame (all subjects in the population) has an equal chance of being chosen.

B. This sampling procedure involves drawing every Nth element from a population.

C. Determine the relevant strata in a population; sample a number of people in each stratum; the number in the sample should be the same as the proportion of the group in the total population. After you choose the strata and proportions, choose the subjects within each of the categories according to random sampling methods.

D. Divide the population into groups (clusters); randomly derive your sample from the list of clusters. Sample all subjects in each chosen cluster, or sample randomly selected subjects from each cluster.

E. This major category of sampling is rigorous and requires that every element in the population have an equal chance (a random chance) of being selected for inclusion in the sample.

F. This major category of sampling provides no way of estimating the probability that each element will be included in the sample. With this approach, the results will be representative of your sample only and cannot be generalized to the accessible population.

G. This type of sampling allows the use of any available group of research subjects.

H. A kind of accidental sampling that involves subjects suggesting other subjects to the researcher, so that the sampling process gains momentum.

I. In this type of sampling, the researcher selects a particular group or groups based on certain criteria. The researcher uses his or her judgement to decide who is representative of the population.

J. This is a type of purposive sampling that involves choosing experts in a given area because of their access to the information of relevance to your study.

K. This sampling strategy is not random and may or may not sample proportions representative of the population. The researcher makes a decision, based on judgement, about the best type of sample for the study. Then the researcher decides what the strata are, depending on the variables that might affect the dependent variable being investigated. Thus, the researcher is aiming for more control than is possible with accidental, or convenience, sampling.

L. The type of sampling used in Grounded theory studies based on emerging theoretical categories in the analysis.

Answers to be found at the back of the book.

Reference

Wilson, H. (1993). *Introducing Research in Nursing,* 2nd ed. Menlo Park, CA: Addison-Wesley.

Evaluating Psychosocial Measurement Instruments

74

In Level 2 and Level 3 studies specific **variables** are defined in the research questions and **hypotheses**. As you critique these studies or as you plan your own research, you should be aware of the ideal qualities of a measurement instrument.

Directions

Read the studies suggested in the references that follow this exercise.

Discussion Guidelines

Discuss the following questions with a group of colleagues or fellow students.

ASSESSMENT OF THEORETICAL QUALITY

1. Is the measurement congruent with the variable to be measured? Is it **valid**?

ASSESSMENT OF PSYCHOMETRIC QUALITIES

2. What are the types and levels of **reliability**?
3. What are the types and levels of **validity**?

ASSESSMENT OF PRACTICAL QUALITIES

4. Does the use of the instrument seem feasible within the particular research plan?
5. Does the measurement instrument or approach to the study respondents seem acceptable?

References

Champion, L. C. (1993). Instrument refinement for breast cancer screening behaviors. *Nursing Research, 42*(3), 139–143.

Hogan, N. S., & Balk, D. E. (1990). Adolescent reactions to sibling death: Perceptions of mothers, fathers, and teenagers. *Nursing Research, 39*(2), 103–107.

Janson-Bjerklie, S., Ferketich, S., & Benner, P. (1993). Predicting the outcomes of living with asthma. *Research in Nursing and Health, 16*(4), 241–250.

Kim, K. K., Horan, M. L., Gendler, P., & Patel, M. (1991). Development and evaluation of the osteo-porosis health belief scale. *Research in Nursing and Health, 14*(14), 155–163.

Muller, M. E. (1993). Development of the prenatal attachment inventory. *Western Journal of Nursing Research, 15*(2), 199–215.

Selecting a Suitable Instrument

Although many nurse investigators develop their own instruments, many good instruments are available to test many different concepts. Often these existing instruments already have been tested for **reliability** and **validity**. Also, if similar instruments are used to measure similar **constructs**, the comparison of findings is easier and more theoretically sound.

Directions

Choose one or more of the resources listed as references. Skim the resource(s) you have chosen and determine if any of the instruments interest you and might be relevant to the research you planned in previous exercises.

Discussion Guidelines

Discuss the following questions with a group of colleagues or fellow students.

1. How would you evaluate the instrument?
2. Is the instrument appropriate for your intended study **population**?
3. Is the method of administration appropriate for your intended study population?

If you find an instrument that has good psychometric properties, you should test it.

References

Clayton, G., & Broome, M. (1989). *Instruments for use in nursing education research*. New York: National League for Nursing.

Mitchell, J. (Ed.) (1985). *The mental measurements yearbook*. Lincoln, NE: University of Nebraska.

Stewart, M., Todiver, F., Bass, M., Dunn, E., & Norton, P. (1992). *Tools for primary care research*. Newbury Park, CA: Sage.

Types of Measurements Used in Clinical Practice-Research

As you work in your clinical areas and think about research projects, you should also be thinking about psychological data-collection instruments that may be appropriate for any study you might read or conduct.

Directions

Have a research topic in mind from one of the previous exercises. Think about the question, purpose, and hypotheses.

Discussion Guidelines

Present your project to nurse colleagues or fellow students and define the following types of measurement tools. Think up a specific research question that could be answered by data generated in each of the types of psychosocial instruments.

1. **Tests of knowledge**

2. **Ability tests**

3. **Rating scales**

4. **Semantic differentials**

5. **Sorting techniques**

6. **Projective tests**

7. **Patient logs**

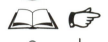

77 ## Planning Research That Uses Biophysiologic Variables

As you know, planning good research requires considerable thinking as well as a review of appropriate literature. This group exercise is designed to encourage your thinking about a specific research problem in nursing that involves **biophysiologic variables**.

Directions

With a group of colleagues or fellow students, choose a problem area that involves biophysiologic phenomena such as feeding alterations, activity and position, patient education outcomes, infection and wound healing, or environmental stimuli. Do a literature search in the area of your choice.

Discussion Guidelines

Discuss the following questions with your group.

1. What is your specific **research question** or **hypothesis**?
2. What are the **independent** and **dependent variables**? What instrumentation is available for measurement of these **variables**?
3. Discuss the **reliability** and **validity** of the available measures.
4. What is the feasibility of carrying out the study?
5. How would this study extend the current nursing knowledge on the subject?
6. What implications for nursing practice does this study have?

Reference

Lindsey, A., & Stotts, N. (1989). Collecting data on biophysiologic variables. In H. S. Wilson, *Research in Nursing,* 2nd ed. Menlo Park, CA: Addison-Wesley.

78 Selecting the Optimal Instrument for Measuring Your Biophysiologic Variables

Lindsey and Stotts in Wilson (1989) discuss several factors that you should consider in making your decision about what instrument(s) is best for your study.

Directions

Choose an instrument(s) from a published research report, review article, instrument-compilation text, equipment catalogue, exhibit at a meeting, or from any other possible source.

Discussion Guidelines

Meet with a group of interested fellow students or colleagues and discuss the following factors and related questions.

1. *Availability*: Do you have access to the equipment you need? Can you possibly borrow it or buy it?
2. **Direct** or **indirect measure**: Can you use a direct measure (which is always better), such as an arterial line rather than a cuff sphygmomanometer for obtaining blood pressure? Which type of measurement is most meaningful and practical?
3. *Single versus multiple measures*: Should you use multiple measures to assess the effect of the independent variable on changes in the outcome variable(s) of interest?
4. **Sensitivity, validity,** and **reliability**: Are your instruments valid? Reliable? Are the instruments sufficiently sensitive to show changes in the parameter being measured?
5. **Invasive** *versus* **noninvasive measures**: Is a noninvasive measure credible? If not, and an invasive measure should be used, is it ethically permissible to use the measure? Will it compromise the patient in any way?
6. *Level of data obtained*: Can you find a measurement that yields **interval-level data**? If not, with what level of data will you be working?
7. *Cost*: Is your instrument affordable? If not, is there a source of funds that can assist you such as another researcher, a grant, a manufacturer? What are the risks and benefits for the subjects?

Reference

Lindsey, A., & Stotts, N. (1989). Collecting data on biophysiologic variables. In H. S. Wilson, *Research in Nursing,* 2nd ed. Menlo Park, CA: Addison-Wesley.

Using the Language of Quantitative Analysis

Like **qualitative analysis, quantitative analysis** has its own language. A good consumer of research and quantitative researcher should understand the commonly used terms. Refer to the Glossary as needed.

Directions

Match the definitions on the right with the terms on the left. Place the appropriate letters in the spaces provided.

Terms	Definitions
_____ 1. **Descriptive statistics**	A. A scale that is "ordered"; the numbers assigned to the data have the characteristics of ordered categories. However, there are equidistant intervals between categories.
_____ 2. **Inferential statistics**	
_____ 3. **Measurement**	B. This specifies all the potential measurement divisions into which a variable might fall; includes at least two categories, is exhaustive, and is mutually exclusive.
_____ 4. **Statistics**	
_____ 5. **Measurement scale**	C. These statistics organize, summarize, and present information in a usable, understandable form Examples are frequencies, measures of central tendency, and measures of variance and correlations.
_____ 6. **Nominal scale**	
_____ 7. **Ordinal scale**	
_____ 8. **Interval scale**	D. A frequently used nonparametric statistic. It is used for testing hypotheses with nominal data.
_____ 9. **Ratio scale**	E. Analytic tools that allow you to show that something is more or less likely to occur according to the laws of chance or probability.
_____ 10. **Chi-square**	F. An inferential statistical procedure that can be used to compare two or more groups by calculating an F ratio.
_____ 11. **Analysis of a variance**	
_____ 12. **Critical value**	G. A process of assigning numerical values to concepts under investigation and is equivalent to actual value plus or minus error.
_____ 13. **Normal curve**	H. These statistics are concerned with making inferences about populations based on samples taken from them.
_____ 14. **Scatter plot**	I. This scale has rank ordering of measure, equal intervals between measures, and an absolute zero point.

J. The size of a number in a statistical table that your calculated number must exceed to reject the explanation that differences are due to chance.
K. The most primitive and least precise measurement scale. This scale arbitrarily assigns some number to represent the categories into which an attribute or quality can be sorted.
L. This scale has an inherent ordering of categories, and the possible measures along an interval scale are equidistant from one another.
M. The graphic or visual presentation of a correlation between two variables.
N. A symmetrical, unimodal curve; also called a bell-shaped curve because the greatest frequency of numbers is at the center.

Answers to be found at the back of the book.

80 Identifying Measurement Scales in Nursing Research

 Quantitative research that measures biological and psychosocial variables requires the use of **measurement scales**. It is important that you can identify the appropriate level of measurement for the given variables.

Directions

Read one or more of the referenced materials in this exercise.

Discussion Guidelines

Discuss the following questions with a group of fellow students or colleagues.

1. What are the **level(s) of measurement** used in the study?
2. Is each level of measurement appropriate for each **variable**?
3. Can you think of how to use a more sophisticated level of measurement for the variables?

References

Brooten, D. et al. (1993). A comparison of four treatments to prevent and control breast pain and engorgement in non-nursing mothers. *Nursing Research, 32,* 225–229.

Cox, C., Roghmann, K. (1984). Empirical test of the interaction model of client health behavior. *Research in Nursing and Health, 7,* 275–285.

Laschinger, S. (1984). The relationship of social support to health in elderly people. *Western Journal of Nursing Research, 6,* 341–350.

Mercer, R., Hackley, K., & Bostrom, A. (1983). Relationship of psychosocial and perinatal variables to perception of childbirth. *Nursing Research, 32,* 202–207.

Snavely, B., & Fairhurst, G. (1984). The male nursing student as a token. *Research in Nursing and Health, 7,* 287–294.

Constructing a Frequency Distribution Table

A **frequency distribution** represents one way of organizing a mass of what might first appear to be overwhelming and chaotic information. It involves systematically arranging numerical values from the lowest to the highest and then counting the number of times each value appears in the data. A frequency distribution lets you see what the lowest and highest scores were, where most of the scores tended to cluster, and what the most commonly obtained score was.

Directions

Given the following raw scores, follow the steps, and construct a frequency distribution.

RAW SCORES

100, 98, 100, 98, 98, 98, 100, 95, 92, 92, 92, 92, 77, 92, 71, 75, 73, 50, 65, 77, 95, 88, 82, 71, 78, 79, 84, 82, 74, 79, 83, 81, 83, 90, 76, 74, 79, 62, 94, 77, 81, 86, 75, 69, 82, 72, 90, 84, 87, 85, 80.

STEPS

1. Find the lowest and highest scores or numbers in the data set for which you want to construct a frequency distribution.
2. Decide what the class interval will be and how many classes you will have. These are commonly called the Xs. Arrange them from lowest to highest value. Be sure that the classes of observation are mutually exclusive and exhaustive.
3. Construct a table that has columns for (a) each class, (b) the tally, or count, of how often the class appeared in the data, and (c) a frequency (a percentage).
4. Read through your raw data sequentially, and make a mark in the count column using the familiar method of four vertical lines and then a slash for the fifth occurrence (卌).
5. Put totals for each class in the frequency column.
6. Add up all the frequencies, called the *f*s, and put the total number for each class in the frequency column. The sum of the numbers in that column ought to equal the total size of your sample ($\Sigma f = n$).
7. Complete the percentage column by dividing each frequency by the total number of data items and multiply by 100 ($\% = 100 \times f/n$).

Discussion Guidelines

Now that you have constructed your frequency distribution, answer the following questions.

1. Can you display the data in a **histogram** or **frequency polygon**? If so, display it.
2. Which do you think is easier to read—the table, the histogram, or the frequency polygon? Why?

82 Measures of Central Tendency and Variability

Measures of central tendency help you visualize the general trend of a group of numbers. The word *central* refers to a middle value in those numbers. **Measures of variability** examine the dispersion, or how the measures are distributed. Both are examples of **descriptive statistics** that help summarize the data set.

Directions

Refer to the **frequency distribution** table and **frequency polygon** you constructed in the previous exercise.

Discussion Guidelines

For assistance, use any statistics text or refer to Wilson's 1993 *Introducing to Research in Nursing*, 2e Chapter 10. Answer the following questions alone or with a group of fellow students or colleagues.

1. Is the distribution **skewed** or **symmetrical**?
2. If it is skewed, is it positively or negatively skewed?
3. Is it a **unimodal, bimodal,** or **multimodal distribution**?
4. What is the **mode**?
5. What is the **median**?
6. What is the **mean**?
7. What is the **range**?
8. What is the **interquartile range**?
9. What is the **standard deviation**?

Reference

Wilson, H. S. (1993). *Introducing Research in Nursing*, 2nd ed. Menlo Park, CA: Addison-Wesley.

Choosing the Right Statistical Tests for Your Hypotheses

Most statistical tests used by nurse researchers in hypothesis testing are classified into two types: **parametric statistics** and **nonparametric statistics.** Parametric tests have important requirements and are more robust than nonparametric tests. Within each of these major categories are specific tests. This exercise will acquaint you with a variety of available tests. (For additional information, see Wilson, 1993, or any textbook of statistics.)

Directions

Match the definitions in the column on the right with the terms in the column on the left. Place the appropriate letter in the spaces provided on the left.

Terms

_____ 1. **Parametric statistics**

_____ 2. **Nonparametric statistics**

_____ 3. *t* **test**

_____ 4. **Analysis of variance**

_____ 5. Follow-up **multiple comparison tests**

_____ 6. **Chi-square**

Definitions

A. This test involves pairing a score in one situation with a score in another and is used in a within-subjects design or a matched-groups design. The test may be one- or two-tailed depending on if you can predict the direction of difference between populations.

B. This test is one of the most frequently used nonparametric statistics. It is calculated from the differences between observed frequencies and the frequencies expected under the conditions of the null hypothesis.

C. These tests have three important requirements: (1) they involve the estimation of at least one parameter, (2) they require measurements on at least an interval-level measurement scale, and (3) they involve the assumption that the variables are normally distributed (according to a bell-shaped curve) in the population, suggesting that a sample/size of at least 20 scores per cell is essential.

D. This is an inferential statistical procedure that can compare the mean scores of two or more groups. To use this test, you calculate the *F* ratio and check the value of that statistic against a table of F values for its statistical significance; you calculate the variability between groups and within groups. If the between-groups variance is large relative to the within-groups variance, the F ratio is large and the null hypothesis is rejected.

E. This statistic (1) can be used with nominal and ordinal measurements, and (2) can be used when the sample size is small and there is no way to assume that the scores follow a bell-shaped curve or normal distribution.

F. These tests help the investigator locate exactly where the significant difference lies after a significant F ratio has been obtained. For example, if you compare three groups and obtain an F ratio that is significant enough to reject the null hypothesis of equal means, you still do not know which of the means are different from the others.

Answers to be found at the back of the book.

Steps in Using Inferential Statistics to Test Hypotheses

When you decide your research requires the testing of **hypothesis**(es), you proceed through some specific logical steps.

Directions

Part A: Put in order the steps in using **inferential statistics** to test hypotheses.
Part B: In the spaces provided on the left, write in order the steps in using inferential statistics. Then indicate by number which statement describes each step.

Part A

Correct Order   ### Incorrect Order

1. _____   A. Select a **level of significance**

2. _____   B. Choose **the right statistical test**

3. _____   C. State the **null hypotheses**

4. _____   D. Look up a **test significance** in a table.

Part B

**Steps in Using
Inferential Statistics
to Test Hypotheses**   **Statements**

1. _____   1. To do this you need to know the name of the test performed, the **degrees of freedom**, and the **confidence level** of the test statistics for whatever degree of freedom you choose.

2. _____   2. First you choose the major category of either **parametric** or **nonparametric statistical** tests, depending on the requirements of each (see Wilson, 1993, Chapter 10). Then you choose the appropriate specific test for your study.

3. _____   3. You make a statement that no difference exists between the **populations** being compared. This is essentially a statement that explains a study's results as being due only to chance factors or **sampling error**.

4. _____

4. When you select this, you are selecting a **probability** that tells you how unlikely the sample data must be before you can reject the null hypotheses.

Answers to be found at back of book.

Reference

Wilson, H. S. (1993). *Introducing Research in Nursing,* 2nd ed. Menlo Park, CA: Addison-Wesley.

85 ## Qualitative Research Methods

Different methods are used in **qualitative research**. These methods have derived from disciplines other than nursing, and as such, reveal the distinct perspectives of those disciplines. If you choose to do qualitative research, it is important that you understand the philosophical perspective of your method of choice.

Directions

Match each qualitative research method with a description listed below.

Grounded Theory

Hermeneutics

Ethnography

Esthetic Inquiry

Phenomenology

Case Study

1. _____ A method used to describe a cultural group or to describe a phenomenon associated with a cultural group. This method, which uses primarily participant observation and unstructured interviews, is based on the assumption that culture is learned and shared among members of a group and as such, may be described and understood. This method derives from anthropology.

2. _____ A research method developed for the purpose of studying social phenomena from the perspective of symbolic interactionism. This method, designed to generate theory, provides a means for describing the social psychological processes that people develop to assist in making sense of their worlds. This method derives from sociology.

3. _____ A method of direct inquiry in which in-depth interviewing provides insight into the lived experience. Writing and rewriting are an essential part of the process of reflection. This method derives from the philosophy of Husserl.

4. _____ An approach appropriate for the study of human action. Using existential understanding and a system of interpretation, this strategy provides a means for arriving at a deeper understanding of human existence through attention to the nature of language and meaning. This method derives from the philosophy of Heidegger.

5. _____ A method of investigating the "particular" involving an intensive examination of an individual, a program, an institution, or a community. This technique aids in understanding problems, needs, wishes, goals. This method derives from law and political science.

6. _____ A method of utilizing such techniques as photography and literature to promote communication and generate data by eliciting participant responses. This approach is sometimes used with other methods for a fuller understanding of the phenomena under investigation. This method derives from esthetics including art and literature.

References

Allen, M. N., & Jensen, L. (1990). Hermeneutical inquiry meaning and scopy. *Western Journal of Nursing Research*, 12241–253.

Bowers, B. J. (1989). Grounded theory. In B. Sarter (Ed.), *Paths to knowledge* (pp. 33–59). NLN Publications.

Hutchinson, S. (1990). The case study approach. In L. Moody (Ed.), *Advancing theory for nursing science through research* (pp. 177–213). Newbury Park, CA: Sage Publications.

Magilvy, J. K., Congdon, J. G., Nelson, J. P., & Craig, C. (1992). Visions of rural aging: Use of photographic method in gerontological research. *The Gerontologist, 32*, 253–257.

Morse, J. (Ed.) (1992). *Qualitative health research.* Newbury Park, CA: Sage Publications.

Munhall, P. (1993). *Nursing research, A qualitative perspective.* NY: NLN Publications.

Wilson, H., & Hutchinson, S. (1991). Triangulation of qualitative methods: Heideggerian hermeneutics and grounded theory. *Qualitative Health Research, 1*(2), 263–276.

Adapted from: JoAnne Weiss, MSN, ARNP
                 Doctoral Student
                 College of Nursing
                 University of Florida

A Fieldwork Experience

Field researchers generally believe one cannot really appreciate the nature of fieldwork unless you experience it. This exercise offers you an opportunity to get a feel for fieldwork.

Directions

Visit an environment that is totally alien to you; for example, a health spa, a country-western bar, a primary care clinic, or an opera. Take notes on what you observe for 2 hours. At the end of the observation time code your data into categories.

Discussion Guidelines

Discuss the following questions with a group of fellow students or colleagues who have gone to the same or a different setting.

1. How did you feel in the role of field researcher? What other feelings did you have during the experience?

2. Which of the observed behaviors did you not understand?

3. What patterns did you see?

4. What categories of behavior could you identify?

5. What methodological notes would you write?

6. What difficulties did you have?

7. What was most interesting to you?

8. What new insights did you gain?

Stages of Field Research

Although **fieldwork** must be flexible so that the researcher can define the world from the perspective of those being studied, there are stages of fieldwork that are present in any situation.

Directions

The five stages of fieldwork are listed on the left. First, put the *stages of fieldwork* into the *correct order* as they occur during research by writing their names in the spaces provided to the right of the numbers. Then match the *description of the stages of fieldwork* with the correct stage by putting the appropriate letter to the left of each number.

Stages of Fieldwork	Correct Order	Description of the Stages of Fieldwork
Gaining entrée and access	____ 1. _____	A. Based on the nature of the study, the researcher decides if he or she will be a complete participant, a participant as observer, an observer as participant, or a complete observer.
Collecting and recording data	____ 2. _____	
Leaving the field	____ 3. _____	
Locating the field	____ 4. _____	B. The researcher gracefully withdraws from the study setting. Problems that may have developed are addressed, entrée bargains are reappraised, and personal relationships are resolved.
Bargaining for a role	____ 5. _____	
		C. Appraise the suitability of the setting to determine if it will yield data bearing on the purpose or research question that focuses the study.
		D. The researcher records the ongoing experiences of the participants while interviewing and being a participant observer.

E. During this stage, you obtain permission from "gatekeepers" to do your study, and you build rapport and trust with your informants so they begin to share information with you.

Answers to be found at the back of the book.

Strategies in Field Research

Field research requires feasibility, ingenuity, creativity, and ultimately analytic rigor. This exercise is designed to let you work with a group in planning strategies to solve potential problems in the field.

Directions

Read the following vignette.

You want to study a group of patients who have been disfigured by burns or surgery. You wonder how they cope with their disfigurement, what they see as their most difficult problems, and what phases they go through as they are forced to live with the disfigurement.

Discussion Guidelines

Discuss the following questions with a group of fellow students or colleagues.

1. How will you find these people? How will you present your study to (a) the gate-keepers and (b) the informants?
2. How will you collect your data? What will you do first, second, and so forth?
3. If you interview, how many people should you interview? For how long? How often?
4. What ethical problems, if any, do you anticipate?
5. What do you have to offer these people (reciprocity)?
6. How do you feel about doing this study?

Learning to Do Analytic Induction

In **analytic induction** the analyst attempts to search for **concepts** and **propositions** in the **data** that apply to all cases of a question under analysis. This approach assumes the careful consideration of all analytic evidence, the intensive analysis of individual cases, and the comparison of cases to one another.

Directions

Get out your **field notes** from a prior exercise and read them several times. Copy your field notes and give a copy to fellow classmates or colleagues.

Discussion Guidelines

Answer for yourself or discuss in a group the following questions (Lofland, 1971).

1. What are the characteristics of what is occurring in your data? What forms does it assume? What are its variations?
2. What are the conditions that preceded its occurrence, and what variations exist in them?
3. What are the consequences of the discovered social phenomenon?

After you answer these practical questions, go through the following steps (alone or in your group) of analytic induction (Denzin, 1970).

1. What is the study problem?
2. Identify general **categories** about what is occurring. Formulate hypothetical explanations.
3. Examine cases in the data to see if emerging propositions fit the facts.
4. Search for **negative cases**, and reformulate **hypotheses** (Step 2) based on them.
5. Continue this process until a pattern of relationships or set of propositions is identified, explained, and supported with data.
6. Compare with other groups or conditions to develop an even more abstract and generalized explanatory schema.

References

Denzin, N. (1970). *The Research Act*. Chicago: Aldine.

Lofland, J. (1971). *Analyzing Social Settings*. Belmont, CA: Wadsworth.

Generating a Taxonomy in Research

Taxonomies provide us with descriptive categorical information about an issue or subject. This exercise gives you an opportunity to develop a taxonomy in an area of your choice.

Directions

Choose the focus for your taxonomy based on your research purpose. For example: To describe how nurses function in nurse-physician team meetings; To describe the problems that occur around "do not resuscitate (DNR)" orders. Collect data with audiotaped interviews and/or **participant observation**. Generate a taxonomy by following Spradley (1979, 1980). Illustrate the **categories** in the taxonomy with **narrative data** from interviews and participant observation. Discuss your taxonomy with a group of colleagues. Use the following questions as guidelines for group discussion.

1. Is the taxonomy credible?
2. Is the taxonomy complete? If not, what is missing?
3. Does the narrative data clearly illustrate the categories?
4. Is the taxonomy useful? If so, how is it useful (e.g., does it inform clinical practice)? If not what information would make it useful?

References

Spradley, J. (1979). *The ethnographic interview*. New York: Holt, Rinehart, and Winston.

Spradley, J. (1980). *Participant observation*. New York: Holt, Rinehart, and Winston.

Triangulation in Nursing Research

91

One of the ways nurse researchers can facilitate study of complex human phenomena is through the use of triangulation. **Triangulation** refers to a combination of methods/investigators/theories/data and/or types of analysis used to overcome the biases and deficiencies present in research that relies on a single method, investigator, etc. Six types of triangulation are identified in the literature. Match the descriptions on the left with the letter of the type of triangulation on the right. Letters may be used more than once.

Descriptions

1.___The use of more than one type of triangulation in a single study

2.___The goal is cross-validation in analysis

3.___Uses multiple methods

4.___Uses multiple sources of data

5.___The research and professional background of the investigators is important

6.___Two or more theoretical perspectives are brought to bear on the same data set

7.___To do this successfully it is necessary that researchers have divergent backgrounds

8.___Disciplinary biases should be presented

9.___Strengths and weaknesses of methods must complement each other

Types of Triangulation

A. **Investigator Triangulation**

B. **Theoretical Triangulation**

C. **Data Triangulation**

D. **Methodological Triangulation**

E. **Analysis Triangulation**

F. **Multiple Triangulation**

Answers to be found at the back of the book.

References

Kimchi, J., Polivka, B., & Stevenson, J. (1991). Triangulation: Operational definitions. *Nursing research, 6,* 364–366.

Mitchell, E. S. (1986). Multiple triangulation: A methodology for nursing science. *Advances in nursing science, 8,* 18–26.

Adapted from: Susan Wozniak
                 Doctoral Student
                 College of Nursing
                 University of Florida

PART 5

Disseminating Nursing Research: Intellectual Craftsmanship

✤ Your Commitment as a Nursing Scholar

Information discovered as a consequence of building inquiry into the definition of your professional role can make a difference only if you report your findings, methods, and insights to others who care about them. You can accomplish this goal in a course paper that you revise for publication, in a nursing journal, in a thesis or dissertation, in a book, or by giving a talk at a professional meeting. Delivering an effective speech about your research and producing scholarly scientific writing are not easy. Writing and speaking on scientific subjects, like any other skills, require practice. But working with the theoretical and scientific need not adversely affect your goal of communicating clearly and with good style. Use Exercises in this Part to diagnose your own technical writing problems and apply what you discover about your problem areas to learn to write well.

✤ General Guidelines for Presentations

Whether you are writing a script for a speech, an article, or a course paper, certain basic principles of good writing should be kept in mind:

1. Write *for an audience* or readership and *from a point of view*. Achieving an appropriate vocabulary and tone for your audience is a big step in the direction of clarity, which defines good scientific work. Remember that language can corrupt thought, and plain English has a lot to recommend it.

2. Get off to a good start. Never begin a presentation or article by apologizing. Resist all temptations to procrastinate getting your ideas on paper.

3. Pay attention to your writing and speaking style. While poetry, stream of consciousness, and original use of words are not encouraged in scientific writing, technique and style are still important. In fact, it takes a good deal of creativity to be clear and precise without being dull. Use a good style manual, and try to make your writing style lean, direct, specific, logical, and lucid rather than stilted. Avoid jargon and cliches!

4. Get organized. A lot of novice writers and speakers use what might be called "the buckshot approach." This involves scattering your ideas as diffusely and repeatedly as possible and hoping you will "hit" some of your audience with some of your points some of the time. The result is disjointed, incoherent, disorganized writing. *Work from an outline*. Develop your paragraphs, and carry your reader or listener forward with logical transitions.

5. Read widely and use writing aids. Reading for fun is probably a habit for most writers, but for aspiring writers, reading for style, structure, and substance is probably the most important influence on your ability to write. Also read and refer to good writing aids such as a style manual and dictionary. Ask your librarian for suggestions.

All good writing goes through a phase of prewriting (planning), writing (expression), and rewriting (editing). Use the exercises in Part 5 to get some practice related to each.

Writing Questionnaire

Directions

Answer the following questions about your writing.

Prewriting   Yes   Maybe   No

Do you narrow your topic to a manageable
  scope?
Do you know how to do library research?
  Can you find what you need in the library?
  Do you know how to take notes on your
    subject?
Do you have a system for organizing the
  material and ideas you collect (outline, list,
  or other)?

Organizing and Developing Your Topic

Do you choose a form of organization for
  your paper that helps you deal with your
  main idea? (HINT: Three broad areas you
  can choose from are exploration or analysis, argumentation, and comparison.)
Do you state a thesis you intend to defend
  in your first paragraph?
Does your thesis predict and control the rest
  of your paper?
Does each paragraph relate to your thesis?
Does your conclusion follow from your
  argument and restate your thesis?

Managing Your Tools (Words, Sentences, and Paragraphs)

Diction:
Do you use words that are precise?
Do you define unusual terms?

Yes   Maybe   No

Do you avoid repeating the same word too frequently?

Is your spelling accurate?

If not, do you check all remotely questionable words in the dictionary or use "spell-check" on your computer?

Do you avoid showing off with fancy language?

Sentences:

Are you able to write sentences that are both correct *and* effective?

Do you use a handbook on usage when you have questions?

Do you vary your sentence structure? (HINT: When all your sentences sound the same, your reader is likely to fall asleep.)

Do you link your ideas with words that show the relationships between them (although, in spite of, despite, in addition, on the other hand, on the contrary, etc.)?

Do you use parallel construction when you mention a series of ideas in one sentence? (If this sounds like unfamiliar jargon to you, you may be unknowingly obscuring your ideas with awkward phrasing.)

Do you avoid vague or general statements?

Paragraphs:

Do you clearly state your main point?

Do you solidly support that point within the paragraph?

Does each paragraph consist of at least several sentences and a significant body of information?

Does the main idea of each paragraph lead logically to your next point (paragraph)?

Do you use transitional words and phrases to link paragraphs?

Yes   Maybe   No

Editing

Do your papers go through several stages (notes, outline, rough draft, final copy)?

Do you know how to edit your rough draft?

Do you let it rest at least a day or two?

Do you read it aloud to hear how it sounds?

Do you refine each sentence until it is as clear and simple as possible?

Do you reshuffle sentences and paragraphs until the ideas flow from one to the other smoothly?

Do you cut out anything unnecessary?

Do you check for spelling and mechanical errors (with a dictionary and a handbook on usage, or spell-check on the computer)?

General

Can you complete a final draft that is:

Mechanically correct (with regard to grammar, punctuation, spelling)?

Effective (accomplishes what you set out to accomplish—in other words, gets your point across!)?

Well-organized (you've stated your ideas in such a way that they make sense)?

Interesting to read? (If not, you may lose your reader in spite of your correctness and brilliant ideas. Cultivate a style that is a pleasure to read.)

Discussion

Decide where you need improvement and identify some resources possibly through your local library or School of Nursing and strategies that will help you to achieve it.

93 Learning to Write Well

Writing well is a reflection of thinking clearly. Writing skills improve with constructive criticism, practice, and rewriting.

Directions

Write one titled paragraph on a subject related to nursing that interests you.

Discussion Guidelines

Meet with your classmates or colleagues and take turns reading your paragraphs. After each report, discuss the following questions.

1. Is the paragraph organized? Is there a lead sentence followed by approximately four sentences?
2. Is the central idea clear to the audience?
3. Did the author use the active rather than the passive voice?
4. Is the language jargon free? Is it definite, specific, and concrete?
5. Are statements in positive rather than negative form?
6. Are there any needless words?
7. Are the verbs vivid and forceful?
8. How could the paragraph be improved?
9. Is the title concise, specific, and informative? Does it tell accurately and clearly what the paper is about?

Consider this phase the prewriting phase. Now that you have received constructive criticism, rewrite the paragraph.

Working Quotations in Smoothly

If you want a paper or a speech to read smoothly, quotations must be worked in carefully. Also, remember that you only use quotations if:

1. The material is authoritative and is convincing evidence in support of your thesis.
2. The statement is phrased exactly the way it should be expressed.
3. The idea is controversial, and you want to assure your audience about it.

Directions

Take a paragraph from something you have written and find relevant quotations to add to the paragraph. Rewrite the paragraph including the quotations.

Discussion Guidelines

After writing your paragraph, ask yourself the following questions.

1. Have you inserted the quotation appropriately (e.g., with an introductory phrase such as "As Wilson & Hutchinson discovered, . . . ")?
2. Does the entire sentence make sense to the reader? Is the grammar correct?
3. Does the quotation you chose meet one of the three criteria listed in the first paragraph of this exercise?
4. If, for clarity, you have had to alter the quotation itself, have you added the required square brackets ([ ]) that notify the reader of your change?
5. If you believe you can shorten the quotation without altering the meaning, have you used a series of dots or ellipses (. . .), to indicate that something has been omitted?
6. Have you put any and all *original* "apt phrases" or segments from other writers in quotation marks and credited the source?

95 ## Writing a Query Letter

A **query letter** asks whether an editor of a journal is interested in reviewing your manuscript for publication. Writing a letter of inquiry, or query letter, to the editor of the journal of your choice can increase the likelihood that your unsolicited manuscript will be accepted.

Directions

Write a rough draft of a query letter for journals you think might be interested in publishing your manuscript.

Discussion Guidelines

Review your letter and see if it meets the following criteria:

1. A lead paragraph or two that catches the editor's interest and lures him or her into reading on.
2. A paragraph that tells what the article will be about, what direction it will take, and what it will offer the reader.
3. Some facts, observations, or other citations that back up your basic premise and offer your credentials for writing the piece.
4. Two final paragraphs in which you make a strong statement designed to convince the editor that this is an article that he or she should publish and asking if the editor is interested in reviewing the manuscript for publication consideration.

Rewrite your letter according to these recommendations.

96 Judging Your Own Writing

Whenever you compose a paper, a letter or a research proposal use the following criteria to judge the quality of your own writing.

1. Are your ideas relevant and logical?
2. Is your document organized to make obvious the emphasis, the transitions, and the development of a theme or direction?
3. Have you used good style as evidenced by tone and originality?
4. Have you attended to mechanics such as spelling, punctuation, and grammar?
5. Does your choice of words reflect fluency and correct denotation and connotation?

✛ Answers to Exercises

Exercise 2

1. D   2. C   3. B   4. A   5. D   6. A   7. B
8. C

Exercise 7

1. NR   2. NR   3. R   4. NR   5. NR   6. R
7. NR   8. NR   9. R   10. NR   11. NR
12. R

Exercise 10

1. 7   2. 2   3. 4   4. 3   5. 6   6. 1   7. 8   8. 5
9. 13   10. 15   11. 12   12. 10   13. 16   14. 17
15. 9   16. 11   17. 14   18. 19   19. 20   20. 18

Exercise 13

1. Violation of principle 1   2. Adherence to
principle 3   3. Violation of principle 2
4. Violation of principle 5   5. Adherence to
principle 4   6. Adherence to principle 7
7. Violation of principle 8   8. Adherence to
principle 6   9. Adherence to principle 10
10. Violation of principle 9

Exercise 16

Definitions	Examples of Violations
1. C 2. A 3. B	1. B 2. C 3. A

Exercise 21

1. NI   2. NI   3. NI   4. NI   5. P   6. P   7. P

Exercise 22

1. NI   2. P   3. NI   4. NI   5. P   6. P   7. NI
8. P   9. NI

Exercise 23

1. NI   2. NI   3. P   4. P   5. NI   6. P

Exercise 24

1. B   2. D   3. C   4. B   5. E   6. F   7. E   8. D
9. C   10. A   11. A   12. F

Exercise 25

1. B   2. A   3. B   4. B   5. A   6. B   7. B

Exercise 27

1. N 2. r 3. x 4. $\overline{x}$ 5. f 6. H_0 7. H_1
8. s^2 9. σ^2 10. $>$ 11. B   12. $<$ 13. X^2 14. n
15. α 16. σ 17. p 18. s 19. μ

Exercise 28

1. C   2. H   3. A   4. E   5. B   6. F   7. G   8. D

Exercise 29

I. Grand theory
   B M
   F O
   I Q
   K S
II. Middle-range theory
   A N
   C P
   D R
   J T
III. Abstracted empiricism
   E G
   H L

Exercise 30

1. K   2. I   3. H   4. G   5. J   6. C   7. E   8. B
9. F   10. D   11. A   12. N   13. M   14. L

Exercise 31

Your outline of heads and subheads resemble
the following:
1. Abstract
2. Introduction
   a. Literature Review
   b. Statement of Purpose
3. Method
   a. Sample
   b. Research Design
   c. Materials
   d. Procedures
4. Results
5. Discussion
6. References

Exercise 35

1. B   2. A   3. D   4. A   5. A   6. C   7. A
8. C   9. B   10. D   11. C   12. D   13. B
14. C   15. B   16. D

Exercise 36

1. D   2. E   3. A   4. B   5. F   6. C   7. G
8. J   9. K   10. I   11. H

Exercise 37

1. A, B   2. A, B   3. A, B, C   4. D   5. D   6. C

Exercise 38

1. B   2. D   3. A   4. B   5. D   6. C   7. B

Exercise 39

1. protection for human subjects   2. setting
3. subjects   4. sample   5. procedure for
data collection   6. procedure for data
analysis   7. instrumentation

Exercise 41

I.   A. 2
     B. 3
     C. 6
     D. 10
     E. 13

II. A. 1
     B. 5
     C. 8

III. A. 4
     B. 7
     C. 9
     D. 11
     E. 12
     F. 14

Exercise 47

1. C   2. F   3. I   4. H   5. K   6. A   7. D
8. G   9. P   10. E   11. J   12. L   13. M
14. O   15. N   16. B

Exercise 51

1. B   2. A   3. A   4. B   5. B   6. B   7. A
8. B   9. A   10. B   11. B

Exercise 52

1. L, N   2. N, L   3. N, L   4. L, N   5. L, N
6. N, L   7. N, L   8. L, N   9. L, N   10. N, L
11. L, N   12. L, N   13. L, N   14. L, N
15. L, N   16. N, L

Exercise 53

1. D 2. H 3. B 4. P 5. K 6. G 7. A
8. F 9. I 10. C 11. J 12. R 13. E 14. T
15. Q 16. S 17. N 18. L 19. O 20. M
21. X 22. V 23. U 24. Y 25. W

Exercise 54

1. K 2. E 3. L 4. J 5. C 6. I 7. G 8. D
9. A 10. H 11. F 12. B 13. Q 14. R 15. O
16. S 17. N 18. M 19. P

Exercise 55

1. F 2. A 3. B 4. G 5. D 6. C 7. E
8. I 9. H 10. J

Exercise 58

1. F 2. D 3. C 4. G 5. H 6. E 7. I
8. B 9. A 10. K 11. L 12. J

Exercise 73

1. E 2. B 3. D 4. H 5. J 6. K 7. C
8. I 9. F 10. A 11. G 12. L

Exercise 79

1. C 2. H 3. G 4. E 5. B 6. K 7. A
8. L 9. I 10. D 11. F 12. J 13. N 14. M

Exercise 83

1. C 2. E 3. A 4. D 5. F 6. B

Exercise 84

Part A *Part B*
1. C   1. State the null hypothesis=3

2. A   2. Select a level of significance=4
3. D   3. Look up a test significance in a
          table=1
4. B   4. Choose   the   right   statistical
          test=2

Exercise 85

1. ethnography   2. grounded theory
3. phenomenology   4. hermeneutics
5. case study   6. esthetic inquiry

Exercise 87

Correct order
C   1. Locating the Field
E   2. Gaining Entree and Access
A   3. Bargaining for a Role
D   4. Collecting and Recording Data
B   5. Leaving the Field

Exercise 91

1. F   2. E   3. D   4. C   5. A   6. B   7. A
8. A   9. D

COMMONLY USED STATISTICAL TABLES

TABLE A. THE *t* DISTRIBUTION

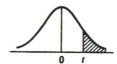

df	$t_{.10}$	$t_{.05}$	$t_{.025}$	$t_{.01}$	$t_{.005}$
1	3.078	6.3138	12.706	31.821	63.657
2	1.886	2.9200	4.3027	6.965	9.9248
3	1.638	2.3534	3.1825	4.541	5.8409
4	1.533	2.1318	2.7764	3.747	4.6041
5	1.476	2.0150	2.5706	3.365	4.0321
6	1.440	1.9432	2.4469	3.143	3.7074
7	1.415	1.8946	2.3646	2.998	3.4995
8	1.397	1.8595	2.3060	2.896	3.3554
9	1.383	1.8331	2.2622	2.821	3.2498
10	1.372	1.8125	2.2281	2.764	3.1693
11	1.363	1.7959	2.2010	2.718	3.1058
12	1.356	1.7823	2.1788	2.681	3.0545
13	1.350	1.7709	2.1604	2.650	3.0123
14	1.345	1.7613	2.1448	2.624	2.9768
15	1.341	1.7530	2.1315	2.602	2.9467
16	1.337	1.7459	2.1199	2.583	2.9208
17	1.333	1.7396	2.1098	2.567	2.8982
18	1.330	1.7341	2.1009	2.552	2.8784
19	1.328	1.7291	2.0930	2.539	2.8609
20	1.325	1.7247	2.0860	2.528	2.8453

TABLE A. CONTINUED

df	$t_{.10}$	$t_{.05}$	$t_{.025}$	$t_{.01}$	$t_{.005}$
21	1.323	1.7207	2.0796	2.518	2.8314
22	1.321	1.7171	2.0739	2.508	2.8188
23	1.319	1.7139	2.0687	2.500	2.8073
24	1.318	1.7109	2.0639	2.492	2.7969
25	1.316	1.7081	2.0595	2.485	2.7874
26	1.315	1.7056	2.0555	2.479	2.7787
27	1.314	1.7033	2.0518	2.473	2.7707
28	1.313	1.7011	2.0484	2.467	2.7633
29	1.311	1.6991	2.0452	2.462	2.7564
30	1.310	1.6973	2.0423	2.457	2.7500
35	1.3062	1.6896	2.0301	2.438	2.7239
40	1.3031	1.6839	2.0211	2.423	2.7045
45	1.3007	1.6794	2.0141	2.412	2.6896
50	1.2987	1.6759	2.0086	2.403	2.6778
60	1.2959	1.6707	2.0003	2.390	2.6603
70	1.2938	1.6669	1.9945	2.381	2.6480
80	1.2922	1.6641	1.9901	2.374	2.6388
90	1.2910	1.6620	1.9867	2.368	2.6316
100	1.2901	1.6602	1.9840	2.364	2.6260
120	1.2887	1.6577	1.9799	2.358	2.6175
140	1.2876	1.6558	1.9771	2.353	2.6114
160	1.2869	1.6545	1.9749	2.350	2.6070
180	1.2863	1.6534	1.9733	2.347	2.6035
200	1.2858	1.6525	1.9719	2.345	2.6006
∞	1.282	1.645	1.96	2.326	2.576

SOURCE: From *Documenta Geigy, Scientific Tables,* 7th Edition, 1970, pp. 32–35. Courtesy of Ciba-Geigy Limited, Basle, Switzerland.

TABLE B. THE STANDARD NORMAL DISTRIBUTION

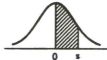

z	.00	.01	.02	.03	.04	.05	.06	.07	.08	.09
.0	.0000	.0040	.0080	.0120	.0160	.0199	.0239	.0279	.0319	.0359
.1	.0398	.0438	.0478	.0517	.0557	.0596	.0636	.0675	.0714	.0753
.2	.0793	.0832	.0871	.0910	.0948	.0987	.1026	.1064	.1103	.1141
.3	.1179	.1217	.1255	.1293	.1331	.1368	.1406	.1443	.1480	.1517
.4	.1554	.1591	.1628	.1664	.1700	.1736	.1772	.1808	.1844	.1879
.5	.1915	.1950	.1985	.2019	.2054	.2088	.2123	.2157	.2190	.2224
.6	.2257	.2291	.2324	.2357	.2389	.2422	.2454	.2486	.2517	.2549
.7	.2580	.2611	.2642	.2673	.2704	.2734	.2764	.2794	.2823	.2852
.8	.2881	.2910	.2939	.2967	.2995	.3023	.3051	.3078	.3106	.3133
.9	.3159	.3186	.3212	.3238	.3264	.3289	.3315	.3340	.3365	.3389
1.0	.3413	.3438	.3461	.3485	.3508	.3531	.3554	.3577	.3599	.3621
1.1	.3643	.3665	.3686	.3708	.3729	.3749	.3770	.3790	.3810	.3830
1.2	.3849	.3869	.3888	.3907	.3925	.3944	.3962	.3980	.3997	.4015
1.3	.4032	.4049	.4066	.4082	.4099	.4115	.4131	.4147	.4162	.4177
1.4	.4192	.4207	.4222	.4236	.4251	.4265	.4279	.4292	.4306	.4319
1.5	.4332	.4345	.4357	.4370	.4382	.4394	.4406	.4418	.4429	.4441
1.6	.4452	.4463	.4474	.4484	.4495	.4505	.4515	.4525	.4535	.4545
1.7	.4554	.4564	.4573	.4582	.4591	.4599	.4608	.4616	.4625	.4633
1.8	.4641	.4649	.4656	.4664	.4671	.4678	.4686	.4693	.4699	.4706
1.9	.4713	.4719	.4726	.4732	.4738	.4744	.4750	.4756	.4761	.4767
2.0	.4772	.4778	.4783	.4788	.4793	.4798	.4803	.4808	.4812	.4817
2.1	.4821	.4826	.4830	.4834	.4838	.4842	.4846	.4850	.4854	.4857
2.2	.4861	.4864	.4868	.4871	.4875	.4878	.4881	.4884	.4887	.4890
2.3	.4893	.4896	.4898	.4901	.4904	.4906	.4909	.4911	.4913	.4916
2.4	.4918	.4920	.4922	.4925	.4927	.4929	.4931	.4932	.4934	.4936
2.5	.4938	.4940	.4941	.4943	.4945	.4946	.4948	.4949	.4951	.4952
2.6	.4953	.4955	.4956	.4957	.4959	.4960	.4961	.4962	.4963	.4964
2.7	.4965	.4966	.4967	.4968	.4969	.4970	.4971	.4972	.4973	.4974
2.8	.4974	.4975	.4976	.4977	.4977	.4978	.4979	.4979	.4980	.4981
2.9	.4981	.4982	.4982	.4983	.4984	.4984	.4985	.4985	.4986	.4986
3.0	.4987	.4987	.4987	.4988	.4988	.4989	.4989	.4989	.4990	.4990

SOURCE: From John E. Freund and Frank J. Williams, *Elementary Business Statistics: The Modern Approach*, 2nd Edition, © 1972, p. 473. Reprinted by permission of Prentice-Hall, Inc., Englewood Cliffs, New Jersey.

TABLE C. THE F DISTRIBUTION (α = 0.05)

Denominator Degrees of Freedom	Numerator Degrees of Freedom																		
	1	2	3	4	5	6	7	8	9	10	12	15	20	24	30	40	60	120	∞
1	161.4	199.5	215.7	224.6	230.2	234.0	236.8	238.9	240.5	241.9	243.9	245.9	248.0	249.1	250.1	251.1	252.2	253.3	254.3
2	18.51	19.00	19.16	19.25	19.30	19.33	19.35	19.37	19.38	19.40	19.41	19.43	19.45	19.45	19.46	19.47	19.48	19.49	19.50
3	10.13	9.55	9.28	9.12	9.01	8.94	8.89	8.85	8.81	8.79	8.74	8.70	8.66	8.64	8.62	8.59	8.57	8.55	8.53
4	7.71	6.94	6.59	6.39	6.26	6.16	6.09	6.04	6.00	5.96	5.91	5.86	5.80	5.77	5.75	5.72	5.69	5.66	5.63
5	6.61	5.79	5.41	5.19	5.05	4.95	4.88	4.82	4.77	4.74	4.68	4.62	4.56	4.53	4.50	4.46	4.43	4.40	4.36
6	5.99	5.14	4.76	4.53	4.39	4.28	4.21	4.15	4.10	4.06	4.00	3.94	3.87	3.84	3.81	3.77	3.74	3.70	3.67
7	5.59	4.74	4.35	4.12	3.97	3.87	3.79	3.73	3.68	3.64	3.57	3.51	3.44	3.41	3.38	3.34	3.30	3.27	3.23
8	5.32	4.46	4.07	3.84	3.69	3.58	3.50	3.44	3.39	3.35	3.28	3.22	3.15	3.12	3.08	3.04	3.01	2.97	2.93
9	5.12	4.26	3.86	3.63	3.48	3.37	3.29	3.23	3.18	3.14	3.07	3.01	2.94	2.90	2.86	2.83	2.79	2.75	2.71
10	4.96	4.10	3.71	3.48	3.33	3.22	3.14	3.07	3.02	2.98	2.91	2.85	2.77	2.74	2.70	2.66	2.62	2.58	2.54
11	4.84	3.98	3.59	3.36	3.20	3.09	3.01	2.95	2.90	2.85	2.79	2.72	2.65	2.61	2.57	2.53	2.49	2.45	2.40
12	4.75	3.89	3.49	3.26	3.11	3.00	2.91	2.85	2.80	2.75	2.69	2.62	2.54	2.51	2.47	2.43	2.38	2.34	2.30
13	4.67	3.81	3.41	3.18	3.03	2.92	2.83	2.77	2.71	2.67	2.60	2.53	2.46	2.42	2.38	2.34	2.30	2.25	2.21
14	4.60	3.74	3.34	3.11	2.96	2.85	2.76	2.70	2.65	2.60	2.53	2.46	2.39	2.35	2.31	2.27	2.22	2.18	2.13
15	4.54	3.68	3.29	3.06	2.90	2.79	2.71	2.64	2.59	2.54	2.48	2.40	2.33	2.29	2.25	2.20	2.16	2.11	2.07
16	4.49	3.63	3.24	3.01	2.85	2.74	2.66	2.59	2.54	2.49	2.42	2.35	2.28	2.24	2.19	2.15	2.11	2.06	2.01
17	4.45	3.59	3.20	2.96	2.81	2.70	2.61	2.55	2.49	2.45	2.38	2.31	2.23	2.19	2.15	2.10	2.06	2.01	1.96
18	4.41	3.55	3.16	2.93	2.77	2.66	2.58	2.51	2.46	2.41	2.34	2.27	2.19	2.15	2.11	2.06	2.02	1.97	1.92
19	4.38	3.52	3.13	2.90	2.74	2.63	2.54	2.48	2.42	2.38	2.31	2.23	2.16	2.11	2.07	2.03	1.98	1.93	1.88
20	4.35	3.49	3.10	2.87	2.71	2.60	2.51	2.45	2.39	2.35	2.28	2.20	2.12	2.08	2.04	1.99	1.95	1.90	1.84
21	4.32	3.47	3.07	2.84	2.68	2.57	2.49	2.42	2.37	2.32	2.25	2.18	2.10	2.05	2.01	1.96	1.92	1.87	1.81
22	4.30	3.44	3.05	2.82	2.66	2.55	2.46	2.40	2.34	2.30	2.23	2.15	2.07	2.03	1.98	1.94	1.89	1.84	1.78
23	4.28	3.42	3.03	2.80	2.64	2.53	2.44	2.37	2.32	2.27	2.20	2.13	2.05	2.01	1.96	1.91	1.86	1.81	1.76
24	4.26	3.40	3.01	2.78	2.62	2.51	2.42	2.36	2.30	2.25	2.18	2.11	2.03	1.98	1.94	1.89	1.84	1.79	1.73
25	4.24	3.39	2.99	2.76	2.60	2.49	2.40	2.34	2.28	2.24	2.16	2.09	2.01	1.96	1.92	1.87	1.82	1.77	1.71
26	4.23	3.37	2.98	2.74	2.59	2.47	2.39	2.32	2.27	2.22	2.15	2.07	1.99	1.95	1.90	1.85	1.80	1.75	1.69
27	4.21	3.35	2.96	2.73	2.57	2.46	2.37	2.31	2.25	2.20	2.13	2.06	1.97	1.93	1.88	1.84	1.79	1.73	1.67
28	4.20	3.34	2.95	2.71	2.56	2.45	2.36	2.29	2.24	2.19	2.12	2.04	1.96	1.91	1.87	1.82	1.77	1.71	1.65
29	4.18	3.33	2.93	2.70	2.55	2.43	2.35	2.28	2.22	2.18	2.10	2.03	1.94	1.90	1.85	1.81	1.75	1.70	1.64
30	4.17	3.32	2.92	2.69	2.53	2.42	2.33	2.27	2.21	2.16	2.09	2.01	1.93	1.89	1.84	1.79	1.74	1.68	1.62
40	4.08	3.23	2.84	2.61	2.45	2.34	2.25	2.18	2.12	2.08	2.00	1.92	1.84	1.79	1.74	1.69	1.64	1.58	1.51
60	4.00	3.15	2.76	2.53	2.37	2.25	2.17	2.10	2.04	1.99	1.92	1.84	1.75	1.70	1.65	1.59	1.53	1.47	1.39
120	3.92	3.07	2.68	2.45	2.29	2.17	2.09	2.02	1.96	1.91	1.83	1.75	1.66	1.61	1.55	1.50	1.43	1.35	1.25
∞	3.84	3.00	2.60	2.37	2.21	2.10	2.01	1.94	1.88	1.83	1.75	1.67	1.57	1.52	1.46	1.39	1.32	1.22	1.00

SOURCE: From *Biometrika Tables for Statisticians*, 3rd Edition, Vol. 1, London, 1966. Reprinted by permission of Mrs. E. J. Snell on behalf of the Biometrika Trustees.

TABLE C. THE F DISTRIBUTION (α = 0.01)

Denominator Degrees of Freedom	Numerator Degrees of Freedom																		
	1	2	3	4	5	6	7	8	9	10	12	15	20	24	30	40	60	120	∞
1	4052	4999.5	5403	5625	5764	5859	5928	5981	6022	6056	6106	6157	6209	6235	6261	6287	6313	6339	6366
2	98.50	99.00	99.17	99.25	99.30	99.33	99.36	99.37	99.39	99.40	99.42	99.43	99.45	99.46	99.47	99.47	99.48	99.49	99.50
3	34.12	30.82	29.46	28.71	28.24	27.91	27.67	27.49	27.35	27.23	27.05	26.87	26.69	26.60	26.50	26.41	26.32	26.22	26.13
4	21.20	18.00	16.69	15.98	15.52	15.21	14.98	14.80	14.66	14.55	14.37	14.20	14.02	13.93	13.84	13.75	13.65	13.56	13.46
5	16.26	13.27	12.06	11.39	10.97	10.67	10.46	10.29	10.16	10.05	9.89	9.72	9.55	9.47	9.38	9.29	9.20	9.11	9.02
6	13.75	10.92	9.78	9.15	8.75	8.47	8.26	8.10	7.98	7.87	7.72	7.56	7.40	7.31	7.23	7.14	7.06	6.97	6.88
7	12.25	9.55	8.45	7.85	7.46	7.19	6.99	6.84	6.72	6.62	6.47	6.31	6.16	6.07	5.99	5.91	5.82	5.74	5.65
8	11.26	8.65	7.59	7.01	6.63	6.37	6.18	6.03	5.91	5.81	5.67	5.52	5.36	5.28	5.20	5.12	5.03	4.95	4.86
9	10.56	8.02	6.99	6.42	6.06	5.80	5.61	5.47	5.35	5.26	5.11	4.96	4.81	4.73	4.65	4.57	4.48	4.40	4.31
10	10.04	7.56	6.55	5.99	5.64	5.39	5.20	5.06	4.94	4.85	4.71	4.56	4.41	4.33	4.25	4.17	4.08	4.00	3.91
11	9.65	7.21	6.22	5.67	5.32	5.07	4.89	4.74	4.63	4.54	4.40	4.25	4.10	4.02	3.94	3.86	3.78	3.69	3.60
12	9.33	6.93	5.95	5.41	5.06	4.82	4.64	4.50	4.39	4.30	4.16	4.01	3.86	3.78	3.70	3.62	3.54	3.45	3.36
13	9.07	6.70	5.74	5.21	4.86	4.62	4.44	4.30	4.19	4.10	3.96	3.82	3.66	3.59	3.51	3.43	3.34	3.25	3.17
14	8.86	6.51	5.56	5.04	4.69	4.46	4.28	4.14	4.03	3.94	3.80	3.66	3.51	3.43	3.35	3.27	3.18	3.09	3.00
15	8.68	6.36	5.42	4.89	4.56	4.32	4.14	4.00	3.89	3.80	3.67	3.52	3.37	3.29	3.21	3.13	3.05	2.96	2.87
16	8.53	6.23	5.29	4.77	4.44	4.20	4.03	3.89	3.78	3.69	3.55	3.41	3.26	3.18	3.10	3.02	2.93	2.84	2.75
17	8.40	6.11	5.18	4.67	4.34	4.10	3.93	3.79	3.68	3.59	3.46	3.31	3.16	3.08	3.00	2.92	2.83	2.75	2.65
18	8.29	6.01	5.09	4.58	4.25	4.01	3.84	3.71	3.60	3.51	3.37	3.23	3.08	3.00	2.92	2.84	2.75	2.66	2.57
19	8.18	5.93	5.01	4.50	4.17	3.94	3.77	3.63	3.52	3.43	3.30	3.15	3.00	2.92	2.84	2.76	2.67	2.58	2.49
20	8.10	5.85	4.94	4.43	4.10	3.87	3.70	3.56	3.46	3.37	3.23	3.09	2.94	2.86	2.78	2.69	2.61	2.52	2.42
21	8.02	5.78	4.87	4.37	4.04	3.81	3.64	3.51	3.40	3.31	3.17	3.03	2.88	2.80	2.72	2.64	2.55	2.46	2.36
22	7.95	5.72	4.82	4.31	3.99	3.76	3.59	3.45	3.35	3.26	3.12	2.98	2.83	2.75	2.67	2.58	2.50	2.40	2.31
23	7.88	5.66	4.76	4.26	3.94	3.71	3.54	3.41	3.30	3.21	3.07	2.93	2.78	2.70	2.62	2.54	2.45	2.35	2.26
24	7.82	5.61	4.72	4.22	3.90	3.67	3.50	3.36	3.26	3.17	3.03	2.89	2.74	2.66	2.58	2.49	2.40	2.31	2.21
25	7.77	5.57	4.68	4.18	3.85	3.63	3.46	3.32	3.22	3.13	2.99	2.85	2.70	2.62	2.54	2.45	2.36	2.27	2.17
26	7.72	5.53	4.64	4.14	3.82	3.59	3.42	3.29	3.18	3.09	2.96	2.81	2.66	2.58	2.50	2.42	2.33	2.23	2.13
27	7.68	5.49	4.60	4.11	3.78	3.56	3.39	3.26	3.15	3.06	2.93	2.78	2.63	2.55	2.47	2.38	2.29	2.20	2.10
28	7.64	5.45	4.57	4.07	3.75	3.53	3.36	3.23	3.12	3.03	2.90	2.75	2.60	2.52	2.44	2.35	2.26	2.17	2.06
29	7.60	5.42	4.54	4.04	3.73	3.50	3.33	3.20	3.09	3.00	2.87	2.73	2.57	2.49	2.41	2.33	2.23	2.14	2.03
30	7.56	5.39	4.51	4.02	3.70	3.47	3.30	3.17	3.07	2.98	2.84	2.70	2.55	2.47	2.39	2.30	2.21	2.11	2.01
40	7.31	5.18	4.31	3.83	3.51	3.29	3.12	2.99	2.89	2.80	2.66	2.52	2.37	2.29	2.20	2.11	2.02	1.92	1.80
60	7.08	4.98	4.13	3.65	3.34	3.12	2.95	2.82	2.72	2.63	2.50	2.35	2.20	2.12	2.03	1.94	1.84	1.73	1.60
120	6.85	4.79	3.95	3.48	3.17	2.96	2.79	2.66	2.56	2.47	2.34	2.19	2.03	1.95	1.86	1.76	1.66	1.53	1.38
∞	6.63	4.61	3.78	3.32	3.02	2.80	2.64	2.51	2.41	2.32	2.18	2.04	1.88	1.79	1.70	1.59	1.47	1.32	1.00

TABLE D. THE CHI-SQUARED DISTRIBUTION

df	$\chi^2_{.005}$	$\chi^2_{.025}$	$\chi^2_{.05}$	$\chi^2_{.90}$	$\chi^2_{.95}$	$\chi^2_{.975}$	$\chi^2_{.99}$	$\chi^2_{.995}$
1	.0000393	.000982	.00393	2.706	3.841	5.024	6.635	7.879
2	.0100	.0506	.103	4.605	5.991	7.378	9.210	10.597
3	0.717	.216	.352	6.251	7.815	9.348	11.345	12.838
4	.207	.484	.711	7.779	9.488	11.143	13.277	14.860
5	.412	.831	1.145	9.236	11.070	12.832	15.086	16.750
6	.676	1.237	1.635	10.645	12.592	14.449	16.812	18.548
7	.989	1.690	2.167	12.017	14.067	16.013	18.475	20.278
8	1.344	2.180	2.733	13.362	15.507	17.535	20.090	21.955
9	1.735	2.700	3.325	14.684	16.919	19.023	21.666	23.589
10	2.156	3.247	3.940	15.987	18.307	20.483	23.209	25.188
11	2.603	3.816	4.575	17.275	19.675	21.920	24.725	26.757
12	3.074	4.404	5.226	18.549	21.026	23.336	26.217	28.300
13	3.565	5.009	5.892	19.812	22.362	24.736	27.688	29.819
14	4.075	5.629	6.571	21.064	23.685	26.119	29.141	31.319
15	4.601	6.262	7.261	22.307	24.996	27.488	30.578	32.801
16	5.142	6.908	7.962	23.542	26.296	28.845	32.000	34.267
17	5.697	7.564	8.672	24.769	27.587	30.191	33.409	35.718
18	6.265	8.231	9.390	25.989	28.869	31.526	34.805	37.156
19	6.844	8.907	10.117	27.204	30.144	32.852	36.191	38.582
20	7.434	9.591	10.851	28.412	31.410	34.170	37.566	39.997
21	8.034	10.283	11.591	29.615	32.671	35.479	38.932	41.401
22	8.643	10.982	12.338	30.813	33.924	36.781	40.289	42.796
23	9.260	11.688	13.091	32.007	35.172	38.076	41.638	44.181
24	9.886	12.401	13.848	33.196	36.415	39.364	42.980	45.558
25	10.520	13.120	14.611	34.382	37.652	40.646	44.314	46.928
26	11.160	13.844	15.379	35.563	38.885	41.923	45.642	48.290
27	11.808	14.573	16.151	36.741	40.113	43.194	46.963	49.645
28	12.461	15.308	16.928	37.916	41.337	44.461	48.278	50.993
29	13.121	16.047	17.708	39.087	42.557	45.722	49.588	52.336
30	13.787	16.791	18.493	40.256	43.773	46.979	50.892	53.672
35	17.192	20.569	22.465	46.059	49.802	53.203	57.342	60.275
40	20.707	24.433	26.509	51.805	55.758	59.342	63.691	66.766
45	24.311	28.366	30.612	57.505	61.656	65.410	69.957	73.166
50	27.991	32.357	34.764	63.167	67.505	71.420	76.154	79.490
60	35.535	40.482	43.188	74.397	79.082	83.298	88.379	91.952
70	43.275	48.758	51.739	85.527	90.531	95.023	100.425	104.215
80	51.172	57.153	60.391	96.578	101.879	106.629	112.329	116.321
90	59.196	65.647	69.126	107.565	113.145	118.136	124.116	128.299
100	67.328	74.222	77.929	118.498	124.342	129.561	135.807	140.169

SOURCE: From A. Hald and S. A. Sinkbaek, "A Table of Percentage Points of the X^2 Distribution," *Skandinavisk Aktuarietidskrift*, 33(1950):168–175. Used by permission.

TABLE E. SQUARES AND SQUARE ROOTS

n	n^2	$\sqrt{n}$	$\sqrt{10n}$	$(10n)^2$
1.0	1.00	1.00000	3.16228	100
1.1	1.21	1.04881	3.31662	121
1.2	1.44	1.09545	3.46410	144
1.3	1.69	1.14018	3.60555	169
1.4	1.96	1.18322	3.74166	196
1.5	2.25	1.22474	3.87298	225
1.6	2.56	1.26491	4.00000	256
1.7	2.89	1.30384	4.12311	289
1.8	3.24	1.34164	4.24264	324
1.9	3.61	1.37840	4.35890	361
2.0	4.00	1.41421	4.47214	400
2.1	4.41	1.44914	4.58258	441
2.2	4.84	1.48324	4.69042	484
2.3	5.29	1.51658	4.79583	529
2.4	5.76	1.54919	4.89898	576
2.5	6.25	1.58114	5.00000	625
2.6	6.76	1.61245	5.09902	676
2.7	7.29	1.64317	5.19615	729
2.8	7.84	1.67332	5.29150	784
2.9	8.41	1.70294	5.38516	841
3.0	9.00	1.73205	5.47723	900
3.1	9.61	1.76068	5.56776	961
3.2	10.24	1.78885	5.65685	1024
3.3	10.89	1.81659	5.74456	1089
3.4	11.56	1.84391	5.83095	1156
3.5	12.25	1.87083	5.91608	1225
3.6	12.96	1.89737	6.00000	1296
3.7	13.69	1.92354	6.08276	1369
3.8	14.44	1.94936	6.16441	1444
3.9	15.21	1.97484	6.24500	1521
4.0	16.00	2.00000	6.32456	1600
4.1	16.81	2.02485	6.40312	1681
4.2	17.64	2.04939	6.48074	1764
4.3	18.49	2.07364	6.55744	1849
4.4	19.36	2.09762	6.63325	1936
4.5	20.25	2.12132	6.70820	2025
4.6	21.16	2.14476	6.78233	2116
4.7	22.09	2.16795	6.85565	2209
4.8	23.04	2.19089	6.92820	2304
4.9	24.01	2.21359	7.00000	2401
5.0	25.00	2.23607	7.07107	2500
5.1	26.01	2.25832	7.14143	2601
5.2	27.04	2.28035	7.21110	2704
5.3	28.09	2.30217	7.28011	2809

SOURCE: From Wayne W. Daniel, *Biostatistics: A Foundation for Analysis in the Health Sciences,* © 1974, by John Wiley & Sons, Inc., p. 382. Used by permission.

TABLE E. CONTINUED

n	n^2	$\sqrt{n}$	$\sqrt{10n}$	$(10n)^2$
5.4	29.16	2.32379	7.34847	2916
5.5	30.25	2.34521	7.41620	3025
5.6	31.36	2.36643	7.48331	3136
5.7	32.49	2.38747	7.54983	3249
5.8	33.64	2.40832	7.61577	3364
5.9	34.81	2.42899	7.68115	3481
6.0	36.00	2.44949	7.74597	3600
6.1	37.21	2.46982	7.81025	3721
6.2	38.44	2.48998	7.87401	3844
6.3	39.69	2.50998	7.93725	3969
6.4	40.96	2.52982	8.00000	4096
6.5	42.25	2.54951	8.06226	4225
6.6	43.56	2.56905	8.12404	4356
6.7	44.89	2.58844	8.18535	4489
6.8	46.24	2.60768	8.24621	4624
6.9	47.61	2.62679	8.30662	4761
7.0	49.00	2.64575	8.36660	4900
7.1	50.41	2.66458	8.42615	5041
7.2	51.84	2.68328	8.48528	5184
7.3	53.29	2.70185	8.54400	5329
7.4	54.76	2.72029	8.60233	5476
7.5	56.25	2.73861	8.66025	5625
7.6	57.76	2.75681	8.71780	5776
7.7	59.29	2.77489	8.77496	5929
7.8	60.84	2.79285	8.83176	6084
7.9	62.41	2.81069	8.88819	6241
8.0	64.00	2.82843	8.94427	6400
8.1	65.61	2.84605	9.00000	6561
8.2	67.24	2.86356	9.05539	6724
8.3	68.89	2.88097	9.11043	6889
8.4	70.56	2.89828	9.16515	7056
8.5	72.25	2.91548	9.21954	7225
8.6	73.96	2.93258	9.27362	7396
8.7	75.69	2.94958	9.32738	7569
8.8	77.44	2.96648	9.38083	7744
8.9	79.21	2.98329	9.43398	7921
9.0	81.00	3.00000	9.48683	8100
9.1	82.81	3.01662	9.53939	8281
9.2	84.64	3.03315	9.59166	8464
9.3	86.49	3.04959	9.64365	8649
9.4	88.36	3.06594	9.69536	8836
9.5	90.25	3.08221	9.74679	9025
9.6	92.16	3.09839	9.79796	9216
9.7	94.09	3.11448	9.84886	9409
9.8	96.04	3.13050	9.89949	9604
9.9	98.01	3.14643	9.94987	9801

TABLE F. PEARSON'S PRODUCT MOMENT CORRELATION

df*	.05	.01
1	.996917	.9998766
2	.95000	.990000
3	.8783	.95873
4	.8114	.91720
5	.7545	.8745
6	.7067	.8343
7	.6664	.7977
8	.6319	.7646
9	.6021	.7348
10	.5760	.7079
11	.5529	.6835
12	.5324	.6614
13	.5139	.6411
14	.4973	.6226
15	.4821	.6055
16	.4683	.5897
17	.4555	.5751
18	.4438	.5614
19	.4329	.5487
20	.4227	.5368
25	.3809	.4869
30	.3494	.4487
35	.3246	.4182
40	.3044	.3932
45	.2875	.3721
50	.2732	.3541
60	.2500	.3248
70	.2319	.3017
80	.2172	.2830
90	.2050	.2673
100	.1946	.2540

SOURCE: Reprinted with permission of Macmillan Publishing Co., Inc., from *Statistical Methods for Research Workers*, 14th Edition, p. 209, by R. A. Fisher. Copyright © 1970 University of Adelaide.

* The degrees of freedom (df) are 2 less than the number of pairs in the sample.

TABLE G. SPEARMAN'S RANK ORDER CORRELATION (SIGNIFICANCE LEVEL, α)

n	.001	.005	.010	.025	.050	.100
4	—	—	—	—	.8000	.8000
5	—	—	.9000	.9000	.8000	.7000
6	—	.9429	.8857	.8286	.7714	.6000
7	.9643	.8929	.8571	.7450	.6786	.5357
8	.9286	.8571	.8095	.7143	.6190	.5000
9	.9000	.8167	.7667	.6833	.5833	.4667
10	.8667	.7818	.7333	.6364	.5515	.4424
11	.8364	.7545	.7000	.6091	.5273	.4182
12	.8182	.7273	.6713	.5804	.4965	.3986
13	.7912	.6978	.6429	.5549	.4780	.3791
14	.7670	.6747	.6220	.5341	.4593	.3626
15	.7464	.6536	.6000	.5179	.4429	.3500
16	.7265	.6324	.5824	.5000	.4265	.3382
17	.7083	.6152	.5637	.4853	.4118	.3260
18	.6904	.5975	.5480	.4716	.3994	.3148
19	.6737	.5825	.5333	.4579	.3895	.3070
20	.6586	.5684	.5203	.4451	.3789	.2977
21	.6455	.5545	.5078	.4351	.3688	.2909
22	.6318	.5426	.4963	.4241	.3597	.2829
23	.6186	.5306	.4852	.4150	.3518	.2767
24	.6070	.5200	.4748	.4061	.3435	.2704
25	.5962	.5100	.4654	.3977	.3362	.2646
26	.5856	.5002	.4564	.3894	.3299	.2588
27	.5757	.4915	.4481	.3822	.3236	.2540
28	.5660	.4828	.4401	.3749	.3175	.2490
29	.5567	.4744	.4320	.3685	.3113	.2443
30	.5479	.4665	.4251	.3620	.3059	.2400

Note: The corresponding lower-tail critical value for r_s is $-r_s^*$.

SOURCE: From Gerald J. Glasser and Robert F. Winter, "Critical Values of the Coefficient of Rank Correlation for Testing Hypothesis of Independence," *Biometrika* 48(1962):444–448. Used by permission of Mrs. E. J. Snell on behalf of the Biometrika Trustees. The table as printed here contains corrections given in W. J. Conover, *Practical Nonparametric Statistics,* © 1971, John Wiley & Sons, Inc.

Glossary

Ability tests: Data collection tools that include intelligence, achievement, and skill tests usually with normative data available for various subpopulations.

Abstract: A section usually located at the beginning of a research article intended to summarize the entire study — including its purpose, design, and findings — as briefly as possible.

Abstracted empiricism: A research approach that focuses on facts in isolation from any theory.

Access: Getting study participants to open up and share their thoughts and feelings with the researcher.

Accidental (convenience) sampling: A type of nonprobability sampling that allows the use of available or accessible research subjects.

Analysis of covariance: (ANCOVA) A statistical procedure used to test the effect of one or more treatments on different groups while controlling for one or more extraneous variables (covariates).

Analysis triangulation: Combining analysis methods to accomplish the goal of cross-validation.

Analysis of a variance: (ANOVA) Inferential statistical procedure that compares mean scores of two or more groups.

Analytic induction: A method of qualitative analysis that searches for concepts and propositions in the data rather than trying to quantify categories.

Analytic description: A qualitative analysis method in which the researcher thinks up original classes or categories by inspecting and interrogating the data.

Anonymity (right of): Protection of the participant in a study such that even the researcher cannot link the participant with the information.

Audit trail: A term used in qualitative research to refer to researcher's notes about decisions made in the collection and analysis of data.

Basic social psychological problem: (BSPP) In grounded-theory studies the unarticulated problem that a group faces in their day-to-day work. This problem is resolved by a basic social process.

Basic social process: (BSP) A core variable(s) that accounts for most of the variation in interaction in a grounded-theory study.

Bimodal distribution: A distribution of values with two peaks (high frequencies).

Biophysiologic variables: Physiological phenomena that vary and can be measured directly or indirectly.

Bracketing: In phenomenology, the process of identifying and holding in abeyance any preconceived beliefs and opinions one has about the phenomena under study.

Case study: An in-depth analysis of an individual, a family, a social setting or a group conducted under natural conditions.

Category system: In observational studies, the prespecified plan for organizing and recording the behaviors and events to be observed.

Central tendency: A measure of a central value or trend in a set of numbers. The three measures of central tendency are the mode, the median, and the mean.

Chi-square: Nonparametic statistical test used to determine whether a significant difference exists between an observed frequency and an expected frequency. Can be used with nominal level measurements.

Cluster sampling: Selecting a random sample of elements that have been grouped into clusters.

Cognitive maps: Visual models or diagrams of categories and relationships in the analysis.

Comparison group: Another term for a control group.

Componential analysis: The systematic search for attributes (components) of meaning for any term used in ethnography and discovered using the ethnographic method.

Concepts: Abstractions that categorize observations based on commonalities and differences.

Conceptual framework: (Conceptual model) A preliminary stage of a theory wherein interrelated concepts offer a framework for conducting research. Sometimes called a theoretical framework.

Conceptual map: A diagrammatic representation of the variables in a theory.

Confidence level: The estimated probability that a population scores within a range of values called the confidence interval; a term used in statistics.

Confidentiality (right of): Means that any information that a human subject divulges will not be made public or available to others.

Confirmability: A term used by qualitative researchers to refer to the neutrality of their findings. Are the Data confirmable?

Confounding variable: Other variables in addition to the independent variable that might affect the dependent variable. Can confuse the interpretation of the study's results if not controlled for in a study's design or procedures. Also called extraneous variable.

Consent form: A written document reflecting an agreement between a researcher and subject concerning the subject's participation in a study.

Construct: Abstract concepts derived from a combination of existing theory and observation.

Content analysis: Method of analyzing qualitative data by compounding the occurrence of specified units of analysis in the data. May refer to manifest content or inferred or latent content.

Control group: Subjects in an experiment that do not receive the experimental treatment or intervention and whose scores provide a comparison against which the scores of the experimental group can be interpreted.

Core category: See also BSP.

Credibility: A term used by qualitative researchers to refer to the believability of their findings. Credibility is similar to internal validity in quantitative research.

Critical Social Theory: The study of existing problems with the aim of questioning the status quo, and searching for alternatives that foster autonomy and responsibility.

Critical value: The value of a statistic that needs to be exceeded in order for the null hypothesis to be rejected.

Data: The information an investigator collects from the subjects or participants in a research study.

Data triangulation: Used especially in qualitative research, this refers to data from several sources, e.g., interviews, documents, and participant observation.

Decision rule: Instruction established to ensure that unusual responses will be scored in the same way for all.

Deductive research: An approach to theory building that begins with existing theory and tests hypotheses deduced from the theory; moves from general to specific.

Degrees of freedom: (df) A concept used in tests of statistical significance, referring to the number of sample values that cannot be calculated from knowledge of other values and a calculated statistic, usually $df = N - 1$, but different formulas are relevant for different tests.

Dense: A criterion for evaluation in grounded theory that refers to the goal of richness and complexity that involves numerous concepts, properties, dimensions, shapes, etc.

Dependability: A term used by qualitative researchers to refer to the reliability of their findings. If a study is dependable factors of change are taken into account.

Dependent variable: The effect or outcome variable that depends on the independent variable; usually symbolized as "y".

Descriptive questions: Research questions about the characteristics of people, situations, groups or settings and the frequency with which phenomena occur.

Descriptive statistics: Methods used to describe or summarize the characteristics of a data set.

Description (analytic): A qualitative analysis method that generates new classes or categories by an active inspection of data.

Description (straight): A qualitative analysis method that uses a classification schema from existing literature.

Design: The plan or blueprint used to get valid and reliable answers to research questions according to canons of science. Also called the protocol or program for a research study.

Diary: A narrative document kept by a study participant and treated as data by a qualitative analysis.

Direct measure: A variable that can be directly measured, such as age or income.

Discriminant analysis: A statistical procedure used to predict group membership or status on a categorical (nominal level) variable on the basis of two or more independent variables.

Document analysis: The analysis of documents such as letters, diaries and records used as data in qualitative research.

Double-blind method: A strategy to lessen effects of inaccurate ratings or responses in which neither the subject nor the data collector knows if subjects are members of the experimental or control group in a study.

Emic perspective: A term used by ethnographers to refer to the way members of a culture view their world; the insider's view.

Empirical (evidence) data: Evidence gathered by the senses.

Entree: A continuous process of establishing and developing relationships with on-site study participants in the field.

Error of measurement: The degree of deviation between the true scores and obtained scores when measuring a characteristic.

Esthetic inquiry: A method of using photography and literature to promote communication and general data by eliciting participants' responses; derived from esthetics.

Ethical inquiry: The study of ethical dilemmas with case analysis. Ethical principles and theories are applied to each case.

Ethics: A branch of study concerned with what is right and good and what one should do.

Ethnographic study design: A qualitative study designed to learn about a culture or sub-culture; typically involves field work or first-hand observation.

Ethnography: The study of human beings as social and cultural organisms; is derived from anthropology; the study of a culture or sub-culture.

Etic perspective: A term used by ethnographers to refer to the outsider's view of the experiences of a cultural group.

Ex post facto designs: A study design that literally studies something after the fact instead of manipulating an independent variable.

Exemplar: A short episode or vignette that captures similar meanings in phenomenologic research.

Experiment: A study design in which investigators randomly select a sample, randomly assign sample members to control and experimental groups, and manipulate at least one variable; can be used to determine cause and effect.

Experimental group: The subjects who receive the experimental treatment or intervention.

Experimental study design: See experiment.

Expert sampling: A type of nonprobability, purposive sampling that involves choosing experts based on their knowledge concerning an area relevant to the study.

Exploratory study: Type of study design used to gain familiarity or achieve insights into a phenomenon. Answers "who" and "what" questions. Also called Factor-naming, Factor-identifying or Factor-searching.

Extraneous (confounding) variable: A factor other than a study's independent variable that affects and confounds or confuses interpretation of a study's findings.

Factor analysis: A statistical procedure for reducing a large set of variables into a smaller set of variables with common characteristics or underlying dimensions.

Factor-isolating questions: Research questions that ask "What is this?" Also called Factor-naming questions.

Factor-relating questions: Research questions that ask how factors that have been identified relate to one another. Answers the questions of "What is happening here?" Also called Association testing.

Feminist inquiry: The study of problems relevant to women. The researcher engages with female participants and focuses on their experiences in context.

Field notes: The notes taken by researchers regarding the unstructured observations they have made in the field, and their interpretation of those observations.

Field research: A term that encompasses the various methods of qualitative data collection. The term "field" refers to the setting where the research takes place.

Field researchers: Qualitative researchers who engage in fieldwork that involves first-hand knowing under natural conditions.

Field: Any social-psychological arena where an investigator gathers data relevant to the area of inquiry.

Fieldwork: Data collection strategies that include observation, interviewing, case studies, and document review; Relies on firsthand knowing under natural conditions. Also called field methods.

Focus group: A group of people assembled to address questions on a given topic, usually a conversational, unstructured format.

Focused interview: Begins with an outline of topics to be covered with every interviewee, but allows freedom to deviate from the prepared agenda as well. Also called a partially structured or semi-structured interview.

Formal theory: (See grand theory)

Frequency polygon: Graphic display or frequency table in which dots connected by straight lines are used instead of bars to show the number of times a class occurs.

Frequency distribution: An analysis method that involves determining how often scores or values appear in a data set.

Grand theory: An explanation of how something occurs under a great variety of conditions. Also called formal theory.

Grounded theory methodology: A systematized method for generating categories and theoretical explanations based on qualitative data. This method has its intellectual roots in sociology.

Halo effect: An observer's tendency to rate certain subjects as consistently high or low on everything because of the overall impression the subject gives the rater.

Hawthorne effect: Changes that occur in people's behavior because they know they are being studied. Was first observed in the Hawthorne plant of the Western Electric Company.

Hermeneutics: The study of human meanings and practices emphasizing the interpretation of lived experience and behaviors from narrative text or stories of research participants; from the Greek word meaning "to interpret". This method has its intellectual roots in the philosophy of Martin Heidegger.

Histogram: Graphic display of a frequency table using rectangular bars with heights equal to the frequency in a particular class.

Historical study design: A study design used to learn about the past based on data that already exist.

Historical method: The study of a past event based on existing evidence.

Human Subjects Committee: See IRB.

Hypothesis: Statement of relationship between two or more study concepts or variables.

Hypothesis-testing research: Studies that test relationships between one or more independent and dependent variables.

Independent variable (IV): A variable that the investigator manipulates; the cause, condition, treatment, or input variable; usually symbolized as "X".

Indicator: Observable data that indicate a concept in qualitative and/or quantitative research.

Indirect relationship: A negative correlation between two variables.

Inductive approach: An approach to theory building that generates hypotheses and explanatory schema from data; Moves from specific to general.

Inferential statistics: Method used to make inferences about relationships and find statistical support for hypotheses in a population based on a sample drawn from it.

Informants/participants: A term used to refer to a person who provides information to researchers about a phenomenon under study, often used in qualitative studies in lieu of the term subject or respondent.

Informed consent: The knowing consent of an individual or his or her legally authorized representative to participate in research without undue inducements or any form of fraud, deceit, duress, or other constraint or coercion.

Institutional Review Board (IRB): A committee established to review ethical issues related to human research.

Instruments: Devices or techniques an investigator employs to collect data. May include questionnaires, performance checklists, pencil-and-paper tests, biological devices, and so on.

Interval level scale: Measures data that rank orders a variable with equal distances between points (e.g. Fahrenheit degrees).

Interquartile range: A stable measure of variability based on excluding extreme scores and using only middle cases.

Interval scale: Ordered measurement categories or numbers with equal distances between successive values.

Invasive measures: Involves penetration of the body or personal space for measurement.

Investigator triangulation: Use of more than one investigator in a study where the professional background of the investigator is important.

Level of significance: Expressed as a numerical value or decimal point; the likelihood of making a Type I, or alpha, error. Also called the "p value."

Level(s) of measurement: A classification system for distinguishing quantitative measures that yield different types of information and are amenable to different analytic operations; the four levels are nominal, ordinal, interval, and ratio.

Lived experience: Term used in Phenomenologic research where the emphasis is on providing detailed description of human experiences; has roots in the philosophy of Husserl.

Mean: The measure of central tendency derived by dividing the sum of the values in a data set by the total number of values, scores, or subjects in it. Also called the average.

Measure of central tendency: A statistical value that reflects the central trend in a set of scores; e.g. mode, median, and mean.

Measurement: The process of assigning numerical values to the concepts under investigation.

Measurement scale: Specifies all the possible values a given measurement.

Measures of variability: The dispersion of a set of scores or how a set of scores is spread out.

Median: The measure of central tendency that corresponds to the middle score.

Methodological triangulation: Combination of methods selected so that strengths and weaknesses of methods complement each other.

Methodological note: Field notes that remind the researcher which methodological approaches might be fruitful.

Methodological study design: A study designed to develop, validate, or evaluate research tools and technique.

Methods (of research): The steps, procedures, and strategies for gathering and analyzing the data in a research investigation.

Middle-range theory: Looks at a specific empirical area and at key variables in depth. Also called substantive theory.

Mobile positioning: Observation strategy in fieldwork in which a researcher moves around in a setting to take notes and collect data.

Mode: The category or class that has the highest frequency. A measure of central tendency.

Model: A structural, pictorial, diagrammatic, or mathematical likeness that represents some aspects of reality.

Multimodal distribution: A frequency distribution with more than two high points.

Multiple correlation regression: A statistical procedure that specifies the relationship between two or more independent variables and a dependent variable.

Multiple Triangulation: The use of more than one kind of triangulation in a single study.

Multiple comparison tests: Statistical tests, normally applied after ANOVA results indicated statistically significant group differences, that compare different pairs of groups.

Narrative data: Textual data usually obtained by taping then transcribing interviews or participants' stories.

Naturalistic\interpretive inquiry: Philosophy of science from the social sciences that focuses on understanding meaning under natural conditions.

Negative cases: Datum that runs counter to the researchers' propositions.

Nominal scale: A scale used to collect categorical or labeled data; arbitrarily assigns a numerical value to represent a category or name.

Nonexperimental design: Study design in which the researcher collects data without introducing any new treatments or changes.

Noninvasive measures: Procedure that does not involve penetration of the skin or personal space for measuring a parameter.

Nonparametric statistics: Tests that can be used with nominal or ordinal data as well as when a sample size is too small to assume that a normal distribution exists in the population.

Nonprobability sampling: A nonrandom sampling technique in which not all elements in the population have equal chances of being selected for inclusion in the sample.

Normal distribution: A distribution that is bell-shaped and symmetric; also referred to as a normal curve.

Normal curve: See "normal distribution."

Null hypothesis: (1) A statement that no difference exists between the population being compared. (2) A statement that there is no significant differences in a study outcome variable (the dependent variable) other than what can be attributed to chance. (3) A statement that there is no relationship between study variables. Also called "statistical hypothesis."

Objective measure: A measure that can be verified by others (e.g., blood pressure).

Observational note (ON): The type of field note that describes the who, what, where, when, and how of a situation, event, or interaction with as little interpretation as possible.

Operational definition: Specification of how a study variable will be measured.

Ordinal scale: A scale used to collect ordinal, or "ordered" data. Ordinal data are numbered or ranked from low to high values, the distance between these values is not necessarily equal.

Outlier: An extreme score in a set of data.

Paired comparison: A data-collection or measurement technique in which respondents are asked to choose between two objects or stimuli based on a specific property or dimension.

Paradigm cases: A whole case that stands out, vividly revealing patterns of meaning in phenomenologic research.

Parametric statistics: Powerful statistical tests that are used with interval level data and normal distribution of a population.

Participant observation: This data collection strategy common in qualitative research refers to the researcher entering the field to observe and occasionally participate in a limited fashion; also called field research.

Patient logs: A data collection tool that is a diary or record of behavior.

Personal note (PN): Field notes about one's own reactions and reflections related to observation in the field.

Phenomenology: An approach to human inquiry that emphasizes the complexity of human experience and the need to study that experience holistically as it is actually lived.

Pilot study: A small-scale practice run.

Population (N): The total possible membership of the group being studied.

Positivist: A philosophy of study that asserts the similarity between the physical and psycho-social worlds and adheres to belief in obtaining objective data through measurement instruments.

Primary sources: First-hand information in historical studies.

Privacy (right of): Enables a person to behave and think without interference or the possibility that their private behavior or thoughts may later be used to embarrass or demean them.

Probability sampling: A sampling technique in which each element in the population has an equal and random chance of being selected for inclusion in the study.

Procedures: The steps taken to collect data in a research study.

Process consenting: The type of consent used in qualitative research whereby the researcher obtains consent throughout the research process.

Projective tests: Used in psychological evaluation based on the premise that unconscious material that is not readily accessible to most people can be projected onto an ambiguous stimulus.

Proposition: Statement of relationship between two or more concepts.

Proxy measure: Measures of variables that cannot be measured directly.

Psychosocial instruments: Measures of psychosocial phenomena; often psychological tests.

Purpose: Specifies the overall goal of a study; what will be accomplished.

Purposive sampling: A type of nonprobability sampling in which the researcher selects a particular group or groups chosen on certain relevant criteria.

Qualitative analysis: The analysis of non numerical data. Often used in field research.

Qualitative research: The study of qualities, patterns, themes and other nonnumerical phenomena.

Quasi-experimental design: A design used when it is not possible to implement all the characteristics of an experimental design such as random assignment to experimental and control groups.

Query letter: Letter of inquiry sent to a journal editor to inquire about receiving a journal article for possible publication.

Questionnaires: A document used to gather self-report information from respondents through self-administration of questions in a paper-and-pencil format.

Quota sampling: A type of nonprobability sampling in which the researcher decides the best, most relevant groups or strata to be included in the study. A quota of each of these strata is sampled.

Random sampling: A sample selected according to one of the procedures for probability sampling that ensures that every element in a population has an equal chance of being included in the sample.

Random sample: (see above)

Randomization: The assignment of subjects to treatment conditions in a random manner (i.e., in a manner determined by chance alone); also know as random assignment.

Range: A measure of the dispersion of a set of scores.

Ranking techniques: A data-collection or measurement technique in which respondents are asked to reorder a set of objects or stimuli based on a specific property.

Rating scale: A measurement instrument on which phenomena are rated on points along a continuum and assigned a numerical value.

Ratio scale: A scale consisting of ordered measurement points with equal distances between successive and absolute zero point.

Ratio measure: A level of measurement where there are equal distances between scores and a true, meaningful zero; the highest level of measurement.

Reflexive: Introspection used throughout a qualitative study to gain insight about the researchers' involvement in the unfolding research process.

Reliability: The consistency, accuracy, and precision of a measure.

Research question: A statement or question that can be addressed through empirical evidence that provides the basis and the direction for a study; a problem that can be investigated using the process of scientific inquiry.

Research design: A set of procedures that tells an investigator how data should be collected and analyzed to answer a study question; a blueprint for the conduct of the research.

Response set: A tendency to respond to items in a similar manner based on irrelevant criteria.

Sample (n): (1) A subset of the population selected as sources for data. (2) Those elements of a population from whom data will be collected and from whom generalization will be made.

Sampling error: The fluctuation of a statistic from one sample to another drawn from the same population.

Scatter plot: A visual presentation of the relationship between two variables.

Scientific inquiry: A process in which observable, verifiable data are collected to describe, explain, and/or predict events.

Scientific approach: The systematic attempt to understand and comprehend the world—particularly its order.

Secondary sources: An account other than a first-hand account used as data in historical studies.

Semantic differential: A type of rating scale typically used to measure attitudes in which the respondent rates an item along a seven-point scale between polarized adjectives.

Semistructured interview: An interview that begins with an outline of topics, but one in which the interviewer and the subject are free to deviate from the agenda as the conversation unfolds.

Simple random sampling: The most basic type of sampling, wherein a sampling frame is created by enumerating all members of a population of interest and then selecting a sample from the sampling frame through completely random procedures.

Single positioning: Data collection strategy in fieldwork in which the researcher observes and records from one location.

Situation-producing question: A researchable question that asks "How can I make it happen?"; a question that establishes goals for nursing actions.

Situation-relating question: A researchable question that asks, "What would happen if . . . ?"; a question in which the investigator manipulates variables to see what will happen.

Skewed distribution: Frequency distribution with off-center peaks and longer tails in one direction.

Snowball sampling: A kind of nonprobability sampling in which subjects suggest other potential subjects to the researcher.

Sorting techniques: A data-collection or measurement technique in which subjects are given a stack of cards with one item per card and asked to sort them into piles based on a specific dimension as level of difficulty or alternatives.

Standard deviation: A measure of the variability of a set of scores; the distance a "typical" score varies from the mean.

Standard error of the mean: The standard deviation of a distribution of means of samples. The smaller the standard error of the mean, the more accurately a sample mean reflects a population mean.

Statistics: A numerical description of a sample. There are two kinds of statistics: descriptive and inferential.

Straight description: Analysis that uses categories from existing literature to organize qualitative data.

Stratified random sampling: Selecting a random sample, after categorizing the population elements into relevant strata or subpopulations.

Study design: Blueprints or plan for conducting a study; includes sampling procedures, methods for data collection, and methods for data analysis.

Subjective measure: Instrument that relies on self-report from study participants (e.g., about attitudes, opinions, behaviors).

Subjects: A person who participants in and provides data for a study; subjects are sometimes designated as "ss."

Substantive theory: A middle-range theory, a theory on an empirical area of inquiry that is the goal of grounded study designs.

Survey research: A type of nonexperimental research that focuses on obtaining information regarding the status quo of some situation, often through direct questioning of a sample of respondents.

Symbolic interactionism: A philosophy of science also called neo-idealist that asserts that the differences between the physical and psychosocial worlds require different approaches.

Symmetrical distribution: The distribution of a set of scores that is symmetrical about the mean and can be divided into two even halves.

Systematic sampling: Involves drawing every nth element from a population to make up a sample.

Taxonomy: A classification based on descriptive categories.

Templates: Cardboard or plastic overlays with holes that allow only certain items being scored on a test to be visible.

Test significance: (significance level) The probability that a relationship between variables could be due to chance; for example, significance at .05 means the relationship would occur by chance five times in each one hundred cases.

T-test: A statistical test used to determine whether two groups are significantly different from each other.

Tests of knowledge: A test used to assess knowledge in a given area or areas.

Thematic analysis: A strategy in phenomenological research that involves recognizing common themes in textual data.

Theoretical framework: An essay in which an investigator summarizes existing concepts, theories, methods, and finding and relates them to his or her study.

Theoretical model: see Model; see Theory.

Theoretical note (TN): The type of field note that describes evolving theoretical ideas for the narrative data in qualitative research.

Theoretical sampling: A purposive sampling approach used by grounded theory researchers to collect additional data based on the emerging analysis.

Theoretical triangulation: Two or more theoretical perspectives are brought to bear on the same data set.

Theory: An explanation of the world; a vision or view on truth or reality; a set of interrelated constructs, concepts, and propositions that present a systematic view of phenomena by specifying relationships for the purpose of describing, explaining, and predicting.

Theory-verification research: Research that is designed to test hypotheses deduced from pre-existing theory.

Timetable: Part of a research proposal which clarifies the overall flow of activities in a sequential statement of operations. Also called a work plan.

Transferability: A term used by qualitative researchers that refers to the external validity of their feelings.

Triangulation: Refers to involving a variety of methods to collect data on the same concept.

Unimodal distribution: A distribution or set of scores with only one mode.

Unobtrusive or nonreactive methods: Data collection approaches that minimize the likelihood that study participants' behavior or response is due to being studied.

Unstructured interview: An interview, either scheduled or spontaneous, in which the respondent is free to talk about anything of relevance to the research.

Validity: The relevance of a measure. A valid instrument measures the concept or construct it claims to measure.

Variable: Any factor that varies.

Variance: A descriptive statistic that examines how scores or values in a data set are distributed.

Index